Teenager's Guide to
Health and Fitness

Teenager's Guide to Health and Fitness

Workout Plans for Sprinting, Distance Running, and Body-Weight Training

Krishna Lingampalli

Copyedited by Michelle Pam Fabugais
Reviewed by Jan Denn Arriba

Library of Congress Control Number: 2013903284
ISBN: Hardcover   978-1-4797-9941-1
                 Softcover   978-1-4797-9940-4
                 Ebook   978-1-4797-9942-8

Rev. date: 02/20/2013

To order additional copies of this book, contact:
Xlibris Corporation
1-888-795-4274
www.Xlibris.com
Orders@Xlibris.com
121145

Contents

I dedicate this book to all the teenagers and adults who take the first step to lead long, healthy lives!

Part of the royalties from this book will be donated to programs to fight childhood obesity.

Preface

Ever since I was a little kid, I had a passion for running. When I was in elementary school, I ran in recesses for fun. In middle school, I really felt the joy of running because I had to run a mile once a week in my physical education classes. However, I was not fit at the time since I had no aspirations to exercise outside of school.

I started thinking about fitness and working out hard as a freshman in high school. Since ninth grade, my passion for running transformed into a passion for fitness. I carried this passion with me outside of the school. Outside of school, I religiously trained several times a week to get fit so that I would be in prime condition for track-and-field season in spring. I qualified for my high school track-and-field team in freshman year. I rose on the team, competing in league meets and regional meets. Noticing the success of my best friend, Michael, who is a fitness fanatic that competes in teen bodybuilding competitions, also motivated me to work out.

When I investigated the causes of youth obesity, I found gorging with poor diet and lack of exercise as the culprits. These bad habits continue when teenagers become adults. It's best to break these habits early.

As I started my journey of lifelong fitness, I slowly learned of effective ways to become and remain fit, which involve watching nutritional intake, getting good sleep, and performing efficient workouts. I wrote this book to share the workouts and tips that I developed to guide others in their quest for health and fitness goals.

Acknowledgments

I would like to thank many individuals who helped me in my journey of creating this book. If it weren't for their encouragement and persistence, this book could never have made it to press.

I give thanks to Kaylie, my track-and-field teammate, who gave me the motivation. She said that I had what it takes to write a concise book on health and fitness. She also gave me tips on what to focus on in this book.

I thank my good friend Michael for reviewing the initial draft. He offered practical, real-world insights into body-weight workouts. He checked to see if the content was accurate that could help out readers.

Finally, I would like to thank my old man. He sat with me for countless reviews and corrections. He also worked with me to organize the content and suggested to make recommendations through the use of tips in every chapter. Without my father, this book wouldn't be as presentable, so I give cheers to him.

INTRODUCTION

Welcome to *Teenager's Guide to Health and Fitness*! This guide will teach you the fundamentals of fitness without any gym memberships or equipment. The guide also provides the basics of nutrition and sleep. You will find practical workouts and meal plans to pursue your health and fitness goals. You do not start a journey without knowing the basics. If you do, failure is set in stone. Think of this book as a compass for your lifelong journey of health and fitness. You can toss this book into your workout bag or keep it on your kitchen counter.

You will reap many benefits on your journey, such as looking good, getting in shape, being stronger and livelier, receiving greater respect, and living a healthy lifestyle. I am pretty sure that everyone wouldn't mind having these benefits.

Some authors write enormous books on these topics that are hard to read because of complicated instructions that throw an average teenager or adult off. Many people give up when attempting to read such complicated books. This book is structured in a way that an average person, who has barely any knowledge of nutrition or working out, can cruise through.

This book is organized into five easy-to-read chapters. The first three chapters will teach you the fundamentals of working out, such as what exercises to perform and the number of repetitions and sets. The first chapter details sprinting workouts along with required stretches and warm-ups. The second chapter introduces basic body-weight exercises for strength training. The third chapter provides an overview of distance running, stretches, and sample workouts. Note that you can choose to work out from any of these chapters to achieve your health and fitness goals. All you need are your commitment and proper attire.

Fitness is only a part of overall health; there are other areas to work on to attain total health. The fourth chapter explains nutrition and rest requirements, such as what to eat and not to eat and how to get a good night's sleep. Chapter 5 has two-week workout and nutrition plans based on what type of workouts you want to execute and your level of fitness. Whether you are a beginner, intermediate, or advanced athlete, the book chapters will tell you what to do.

Many pictures and easy-to-follow steps are included throughout the book to guide you. Additionally, there are valuable tips in every chapter gathered from my years of experience.

After reading this book, you will be able to formulate your own workout and meal plans to fit your lifestyle. It is my goal to help you start and sail on in your journey. So take a leap of faith and flip the page!

CHAPTER 1

SPRINTING

Sprinting workouts are the best things you can do to get into shape. Why? Well, first understand what sprinting is. Sprinting involves you taking your body to top speed or close to top speed in a short distance, say 50 to 100 meters (1 meter is about 9% longer than a yard or 3 feet). Sprinters use tremendous amounts of energy in short periods. Sprinting workouts can go from easy to living hell! I had my fair share of these insane sprinting workouts!

Sprinting workouts are also the most efficient workouts you can do for best results. After starting sprinting workouts, I immediately progressed toward getting in better shape and having more energy and focus.

Sprinting can be done on a track, track-and-field track, park, pavement, or on a clear road. My preference is a school track-and-field track. I am sure that people have access to track-and-field tracks in their local public high schools. Before going deep into the topic of sprinting, let me digress briefly to talk about stretches and warm-ups.

Warming Up for Sprinting Workouts

Warming up before and after sprinting workouts is a must to achieve optimum results and proper body recovery for the next workout! Warming up for sprinting workouts should only be hard enough to stimulate your muscles for the workout. Trust me, you don't want to skip a warm-up and suddenly start your sprinting workout because you will get cramps and pull a muscle if you do so. So based on one's level of fitness, I recommend from one to four laps of easy jogging around the track. Take as long as you need to warm up because you decide whether or not you are ready to start a workout. If you need 15 to 20 minutes to warm up, then go for it.

For sprinting workouts, I recommend performing dynamic stretches as part of warming up. Dynamic stretching gets your body ready to tackle the physically demanding aspects of your workouts. It also helps to increase your ability to perform. Some dynamic stretches I recommend are the following:

- High knees
- Knee hugs
- Quad walks

High Knees

1. Start walking.
2. Bring one knee up to your waistline and attempt to bring it higher as you get better.
3. Bring the other knee up and repeat.

When you are doing this warm-up, bring your feet up as fast as possible. The goal is to get the most number of repetitions of high knees in a relatively short distance. Make sure you go across slowly. Going across quickly or even at walking pace demeans the purpose of this stretch.

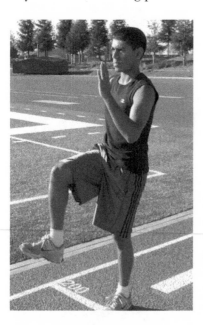 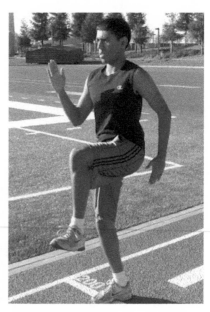

Knee Hugs

Knee hugs are much easier to do than high knees.

1. Start walking slowly.
2. Go across a distance (5 meters at a minimum) by bringing your knees up to your stomach one at a time.
3. Keep your balance and focus on the stretch by going across the track slowly.

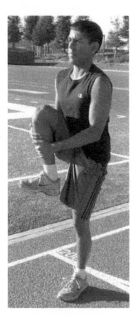 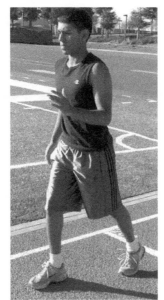 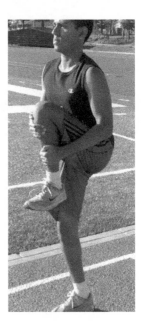

Quad Walk

1. To perform quad walks, start walking, and bring your heel up to your bottoms.
2. Then go forward while switching legs. Bring one heel up at a time.

Watch out! This stretch requires you to have balance.

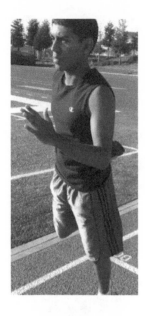
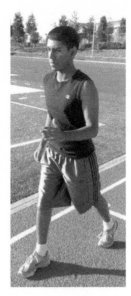
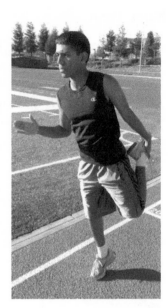

Always remember to warm up!

Tip 1.1: For best results, do your dynamic stretches on the track, and have a distance of about 10 to 20 feet from obstacles.

Sprinting Workouts

Now back to the sprinting topic. There are many sprinting workouts you can do on a track. But what types of sprints are there? To keep it simple, let's distill sprinting workouts into four types:

- Short-distance sprinting
- Long-distance sprinting
- Pyramids
- Relays and game of tag (fun workouts)

Short-Distance Sprinting

Short-distance sprinting involves exerting a great deal of muscular power and joint strength over a short period of time. This type of sprinting has more to do with strength than endurance. A short-distance sprinting workout will not exceed sprints of 200 meters on a track. Remember, when I say *track*, I mean "track-and-field track," like the ones in high schools and colleges. Refer to the picture of a typical high school track-and-field track below. The oval-shaped track is made of four 100-meter segments.

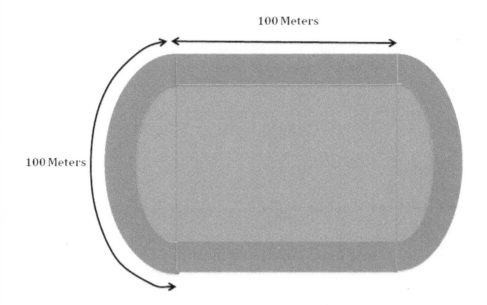

100 Meters

100 Meters

There are several short-distance sprinting workouts as listed below.

* Accelerations
* 2 × 50/100 meters
* 5 × 100 meters
* 4 × 200 meters

Tip 1.2: I do not recommend going 100% all out for a grueling workout because if you do sprinting workouts back to back and all out every day for a length of time, then you won't be able to recover well. Moreover, when you sprint at 100% top speed/intensity, you could get injured.

Accelerations

The first workout for short-distance sprinting is what I call accelerations. This workout is meant to be at a normal level of rigorousness because of the way it was designed. First you need to mark three distance segments of 30 meters each. Use cones at each of the 30-meter markers.

Step 1

First jog 30 meters from first set of cones to second set of cones.

Step 2

Sprint all out to third set of cones in second segment. It is perfectly normal to go all out here because the distance is only 30 meters and you most likely will not hit top speed by the end of the third set of cones (second 30-meter segment).

Step 3

Then jog to the last set of cones. If you don't have cones like most people, use some books at each 30-meter mark.

Tip 1.3: I recommend floating during the first and last 30-meter segments that you aren't sprinting for a better workout. Floating is a type of running where you use your legs much more than your arms when you run. When you sprint, you use your arms quite a bit because they drive your legs forward. So when you float, move at jogging speed. But if you want to jog and avoid the complication of floating, then go for it!

---

2 × 50/100 Meters

The next short-distance workout is sprinting two 50/100-meter strips.

Step 1

After stretching/warming up, sprint 50 meters from a starting line.

Step 2

Walk 50 meters to the second starting line.

Step 3

Sprint 100 meters from the second starting line to the third.

Step 4

Walk 100 meters to the next (fourth) starting line.

Step 5

Then go for another 100-meter sprint. You will have completed one trip around the track after this step.

Step 6

Walk 100 meters to the next starting line.

Step 7

Finally, do a 50-meter sprint, and go to cooldown mode.

Tip 1.4: I recommend doing this workout at 70% top speed for a moderate workout. If you want the rigor of a normal workout, go for 80% of top speed. *And* if you really want to churn some muscle (hard workout), then go for 95% top speed.

---

5 × 100 Meters

Another short-distance sprinting workout is doing five 100s. Translation: you sprint five 100-meter sprints.

Step 1

First you sprint a 100-meter stretch on the track.

Step 2

Then you walk the next 100 meters to the next starting line and wait 1 minute for rest/recovery.

Step 3

Then repeat the process until you complete all five 100-meter sprints.

Tip 1.5: If you want this to be an easy workout, then I recommend going at 70% top speed. Normal workout would be at 80% top speed, and a challenging workout would be at 95% top speed.

---

4 × 200 Meters

The last workout for short-distance sprinting comprises four 200-meter sprints.

Step 1

Go to starting line, and sprint the first 200 meters.

Step 2

Right when you finish the first 200-meter sprint, slow down and walk 200 meters to the next starting line, and rest there for 2 minutes.

Step 3

Repeat the process with steps 1 and 2 until all four 200-meter segments are completed.

Tip 1.6: If you want to go easy, then go at 70% of top speed

If you want to go normal, then hit around 80% top speed. If you really want to go hard and really want to get that body that you desire, then go at 95% top speed for five 200s. No, you did not read that wrong. If you want to go hard, increase the number of 200-meter sprints by one more, and bump up the speed to 95% top speed. The extra 200-meter sprint is vital for increased difficulty because exactly when your body is trying to quit, you make it work for another round of sprinting. Going beyond what your body is used to brings in better results.

Long-Distance Sprinting

Now we will dive into long-distance sprinting. Long-distance sprinting workouts can vary between difficult and extreme. These workouts can take a toll on your body if you ramp up distance or intensity quickly. I remember when I first started doing long-distance sprinting workouts; I would wake up the next day, and all the muscles in my body would be sore. *But* over time, results started showing!

Your workouts need to get progressively harder if you want to continuously make advances. This is because your muscles adapt to the type of workouts you do over a period of time. As a result, the same workouts become easier. For example, think of when you started middle school. Since there was more walking between classes, your lower body got sore the next day. After a few weeks, you were used to all that walking in middle school and your lower body was no longer sore. If you want to get results, then I suggest that you start off long-distance sprinting workouts with easy- to medium-level intensity (this applies to short-distance workouts as well). As you get into better shape and gain strength over time, start doing more challenging long-distance sprinting workouts.

So now let's start off with the long-distance sprinting workouts listed below.

- UCLA workout
- 4 × 400 meters
- 4 × 600 meters

UCLA Workout

This workout was developed by John Smith, a former track-and-field coach at the University of California, Los Angeles (UCLA). This workout is mind-blowingly effective, but at the same time, it is ingeniously insane.

Step 1

Sprint 100 meters forward.

Step 2

Jog (notice it is *jog,* not *sprint*) in the opposite direction for 50 meters. Consider this as one repetition.

Step 3

Immediately turn in the forward direction, and begin rep 2 with 100-meter sprinting.

Step 4

Continue till you get to the end of the first lap of the track, which is equal to one set of UCLA workout. You finish where you started.

Tip 1.7: Recommended intensity is between 80% and 90% top speed because you are going to be dead tired by the end of the first lap. If you have the guts, try going for a second set. One set of UCLAs is crazy enough.

Note that when I mean *top speed*, it is for a given intensity of the workout and strength you have at the moment. In other words, your 90% top speed in one workout can vary from another workout.

4 × 400 Meters

Yes, you can sprint 400 meters, but since 400 meters is a long distance for sprinting, you should only do this workout at 90% top speed.

Step 1

First sprint 400 meters.

Step 2

Then rest at the finish line for 5 minutes.

Step 3

Repeat the process in steps 1 and 2 until you finish all four 400-meter segments.
Since the breaks are pretty long, I suggest for you to relax and drink some water.

4 × 600 Meters

The last long-distance sprinting workout is four 600-meter sprints. "Oh, only 1.5 laps four times? That's not bad!" *Yeah,* if you jog 600 meters, then you will have a relaxing time. But if you run at extreme intensity, oh god, the gates of hell open. After running the first 600-meter sprint, you will feel so exhausted that you won't be able to think straight.

Step 1

First sprint 600 meters.

Step 2

Then rest at the finish line you stopped at for 4 minutes.

Step 3

Repeat the process in steps 1 and 2 until you finish all four 600-meter sprints.

Tip 1.8: I recommend that you run at 80% top speed because of the sheer intensity of the workout.

Pyramids

What are pyramids in sprinting? Well, they are very useful and effective sprinting exercises. Basically, pyramids in sprinting involve distances from small to large to small.

Pyramid Workout

Step 1

Sprint 50 meters then walk 50 meters.

Step 2

Sprint 100 meters then walk 100 meters.

Step 3

Sprint 150 meters then walk 150 meters.

This pattern goes all the way up to 350 meters, but then the pattern goes in reverse. Once you get to sprint/walk 350 meters, sprint/walk 300 meters, then sprint/walk 250 meters and so on until you reach the sprint/walk

50-meter segments. The point of sprinting in this fashion is to really work your muscles. I recommend going at 90% top speed for pyramid sprinting.

Now you may be pondering if there are sprinting workouts where you can have great fun. *Don't worry!* There are a bunch of fun sprinting workouts that involve other people. So since we are on the sprinting topic, let's dive into a few fun sprinting workouts like relays and game of tag!

Relays

The first entertaining workouts I have for you are *relays*, precisely, 100-meter, 200-meter, and 400-meter relays. If you don't know what *relay* means, then don't worry! A relay is where person 1 travels a certain distance (whether it is running, walking, sprinting, or even belly flopping) and then passes an item to person 2, who then travels the same distance and hands off the item to person 3, and so on.

A relay can include many people (typically four in track meets), so it can become an extremely fun exercise to participate. Relays are also fun when two or more teams race. The first type of relay we will cover is the 100-meter relay, more commonly known as the 4 by 100 or 4 by 1. You need five people for a single team: one timer and four runners. The item to use for passing should be a large stick. In real track-and-field events, batons are used; but seriously, how many people have batons? So go with a stick!

In track and field, real relays start at distinct lines on the track, not at regular starting lines. Also, before runner 1 passes the baton to runner 2, runner 2 will already be running to synchronize with the running speed of runner 1. If I explain how to do the relays as legit track-and-field relays, then most people would get confused and would choose to not do the relay. In the revised 100-meter relay, each of the four runners is at the starting line. The first runner leaps into action when the timer says "Go." Then runner 1 passes the stick to runner 2 at the first 100-meter mark. Then from standstill, runner 2 sprints 100 meters to runner 3, who is at the 200-meter mark, and then passes the stick to runner 3. Runner 3 completes another 100-meter sprint and passes the stick to runner 4, who completes the 4 by 100 relay.

For the revised 2-by-200-meter (2 by 2) relay, you will need two runners and one timer for each team. Have runner 1 at the starting line. Then have runner 2 at the 200-meter mark. Once the timer says "Start," runner 1 sprints from a standstill and passes the stick to runner 2 at the 200-meter mark. Runner 2 will then finish the relay at runner 1's starting line.

Tip 1.9: The runner who passes the stick to the next runner should slow down on the side of the track in order to not obstruct the relay if there are multiple teams.

Tip 1.10: Remember, in these 4 by 1 and 2 by 2 relays, start off from a standstill when the runner before you passes the stick to you.

The 4-by-400-meter relay is very challenging and fun at the same time because it consists of four runners who each sprint a distance of 400 meters. The relay total distance is 1,600 meters or close to one mile. Runner 1 completes the first 400-meter lap and passes the stick (or baton) to runner 2. Then runner 2 passes the stick to runner 3 at the end of the second 400-meter lap. Runner 3 then completes the third lap and passes the stick to runner 4, who finishes the last lap and the relay.

Tip 1.11: If you do a relay, then take the next day off to recover because relays take a toll on your body.

Game of Tag

Another fun sprinting workout involves the game of tag. I call it the 50-meter run and fun. The 50-meter run and fun requires two people. Runner 1 attempts to tag runner 2 by the 50-meter mark. On the turnaround, runner 2 chases runner 1 and attempts to tag him or her. At the starting line, runner 2 is behind runner 1. Count going back and forth as one set. Try to do 5 to 6 sets.

What if you do not have access to a track?

Now that we covered everything there is to sprinting on a track, let's go to offtrack sprinting because I know a few of you, readers, will make the excuse, "Oh, I don't have access to a track, no more sprinting for me." Well, guess what? For every excuse, there is a rebuttal. *No more excuses*. There are four types of surfaces you can sprint if you do not have access to a track. They are the following:

- Downhill
- Uphill
- Flat ground
- Curves

Downhill Sprinting

Downhill sprinting is fun, but watch out! It can be dangerous if done in places with moving vehicles. When you do downhill sprints, you go so fast due to gravity that sometimes your own body can't handle the speed you are going at because it is well beyond your top speed. The best place where you can perform downhill sprints is on a road sloping down on a hill with no crossroads so that cars can't come in your way.

Now, the workout I have for downhill sprinting is doing four to five 50-meter sprints all out. Make sure that you have plenty of space to slow down after the 50 meters. To estimate the distance of 50 meters, think of the distance of 100 meters on the track, then imagine that strip divided in half. Then you are all set for estimating distances for your workouts.

Step 1

Start with a 50-meter downhill sprint at 100% top speed.

Step 2

Walk back up to the starting line, and take 2 minutes' rest.

Step 3

Repeat the process till you finish four sprints.

If you really want to push yourself, then complete five 50-meter sprints.

Uphill Sprinting

As for uphill sprints, it gets pretty brutal. The uphill sprinting workout is doing four 50-meter sprints all out. You may think that this workout is the same as the downhill sprinting workout and that the only difference is that it is uphill, but trust me, it isn't. This uphill sprinting workout is at least twice as hard as the downhill sprinting workout. Doing sprints uphill will take the life out of you, but it's worth it because of the results that will follow.

Step 1

Sprint 50 meters uphill at 100% top speed.

Step 2

Walk down to the starting line, and rest for 3 minutes.

Step 3

Repeat the process till you get four sprints.

Flat-Ground Sprinting

Now let's talk about flat-ground sprinting. It is best to do flat-ground sprinting on a level park grass or on some field. Depending on what you could find, you may be limited in flat-ground distance to sprint on. The workouts I have are six 50-meter sprints and four 150-meter sprints. If you have a distance of about 200 meters, then do the 150-meter sprinting workout; and if you have less space, then go with the 50-meter sprinting workout.

Tip 1.12: For the 50-meter sprinting workout, go at 90% top speed for all six 50-meter sprints, and take two minutes' rest in between sprints. For the 150-meter sprinting workout, go at 90% top speed and take two to three minutes' rest in between sprints.

Caution: Be knowledgeable of the ground you are sprinting on! Suppose the surface is grass and there is a small hole you step into, you may lose your footing and get hurt.

Curves

Sprinting curves is really good for a sprinting workout. I will leave making curve sprinting workouts up to you. Just remember to keep the distance to a maximum of 200 meters and at 90% top speed. Also keep in mind the types of curves, such as curves that go uphill, downhill, or both.

nt aspect of sprinting is that you must cool down after
ır cooldowns, go for a nice jog for two laps on the grass
... Afterward, you should drink water and enjoy the rest of

I hope that you are knowledgeable enough to start sprinting and get fit.

To improve sprinting or distance-running workouts, you need to develop muscle strength, which I will cover in the next chapter. Now, on to the body-weight exercises chapter!

CHAPTER 2

BODY-WEIGHT EXERCISES

Body-weight exercises use your body and gravity. They do not require any machines. These exercises strengthen your muscles and help push you to higher levels of fitness. Additionally, by doing body-weight exercises, your muscles will be more noticeable and better shaped, thus enhancing your overall physique. There are numerous types of body-weight exercises you can include in workouts to improve your level of fitness. A certain number of reps are done in a set, and a certain number of sets are done in body-weight workouts. And there is usually a rest time ranging from 30 seconds to 1 minute between sets.

But before we get started, I must remind you that as you include body-weight exercises here and there, over time, they will gradually become easier to perform. If you do the same exercises over and over for a long period of time, then your body will get used to the exercises, and you will not be able to produce quality results. You should change the order of body-weight exercises and increase the intensity every four to eight weeks. People need to constantly shock their muscles in order to make continuous gains.

Body-Weight Workouts

The main exercises that strengthen your muscles are grouped into three categories: upper body, lower body, and abdominals.

Upper Body

- Normal push-ups
- Tricep push-ups
- Tricep dips

Lower Body

- Squats
- Glute-ups
- Wall chairs
- Jumps

Abdominals

- Sit-ups
- Overhead raises
- Scissors
- Planks
- Side planks

I will describe each of these exercises in detail. Refer to the following picture for muscle groups.

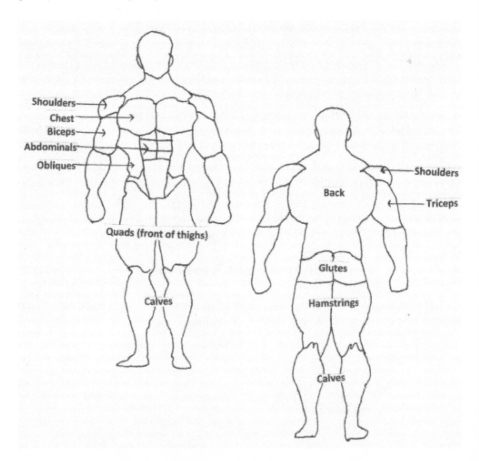

Upper Body

Normal Push-ups

Push-ups are exercises that many people know. They primarily work the chest muscles and use the abdominals as supporting muscles. Perform push-ups as follows:

Step 1

First lie down flat on level ground with your face to the floor.

Step 2

Next make your arms perpendicular to the ground by raising yourself.

Step 3

Then lift your knees off the ground so that you are as straight as a plank.

Step 4

Keep your arms apart a bit more than shoulder width. Make sure that your body is at an angle between 20 and 40 degrees from the ground.

Step 5

Then by remaining straight, bend your arms so that you make an angle of 90 degrees with your arms and neck to see that your upper arms are parallel to the ground.

Step 6

Raise yourself from the ground till your arms are once again perpendicular to the ground. If you feel your chest being worked, then you are doing the exercise correctly.

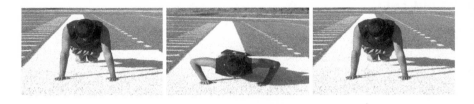

Tip 2.1: I recommend 5 to 10 reps for 3 to 5 sets for a beginner. If you are in good shape, then go for 10 to 20 reps for 4 to 5 sets. For both of these workouts, have a rest time of your choice between 30 and 60 seconds. And remember, one push-up equals one rep.

Tricep Push-ups

Tricep push-ups primarily work the triceps and use the chest a little bit. Performing tricep push-ups is a great way to enhance the appearance of your triceps. You do tricep push-ups the same way you do regular push-ups. The only difference is that your hands are 0 to 3 inches away from each other. So when you do a tricep push-up, your arms will be closer to your body.

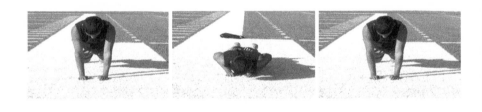

Tip 2.2: If you are a novice, then do 5 reps for 3 to 5 sets. If you are intermediate or advanced, then do 10 to 30 reps for 5 to 6 sets.

Tricep Dips

Another exercise that works the triceps really hard is the tricep dip. A tricep dip is a tricep push-up done backward.

Step 1

First lie down with your face and chest facing up.

Step 2

Keep your body in a straight line, and come off the ground at a 10- to 30-degree angle. Your palms and the heels of your feet should touch the ground and keep your arms as straight as possible. Keep your palms 0 to 12 inches apart. I prefer 10 inches because it puts the least amount of stress on the elbows.

Step 3

Then dip down to the ground by bending your arms slowly till you get around 80- to 130-degree lock in your arms.

Step 4

Next rise back up until your arms lock out.

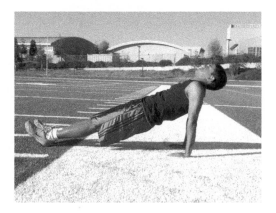

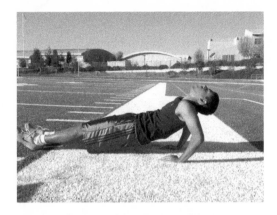

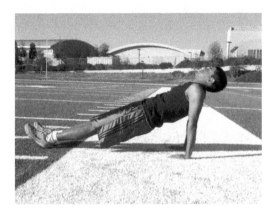

Tip 2.3: If you are a beginner, then go with 3 to 4 reps for 3 to 4 sets. And if you are experienced, then go for 5 to 15 reps for 4 sets.

I set the maximum number of sets to four because of the amount of pump you get in your arms by doing this exercise. Once you get the pump, it's much more challenging to have the correct form. The pump is when blood rushes so fast through your working muscles that it makes the muscles feel very tight and gives a pleasurable sensation.

Lower Body

Squats

Squatting is an exercise that works your quadriceps (the muscles in the front of your thighs) and your gluteal muscles (buttocks muscles) to some extent. Perform this exercise with the following steps:

Step 1

First stand up straight.

Step 2

Then lower your torso down straight until your legs make a 90-degree angle. As you are going down, look straight ahead and push your buttocks out.

Step 3

When you get down to 90 degrees, shoot back up to complete one rep.

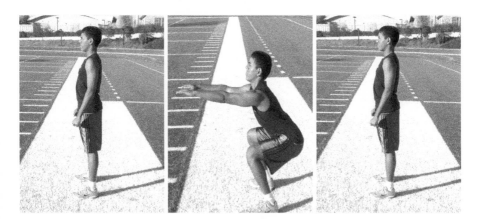

Tip 2.4: Squatting for 5 sets of 10 reps each with 45 seconds of rest time between the sets is perfect for a beginner. If you are in good shape, I recommend doing 10 sets of 20 reps each with a rest time between 45 seconds and 60 seconds.

Glute-ups

Another body-weight exercise that I consider highly effective is what I call a glute-up. A glute-up focuses on your gluteal muscles. A glute-up can be performed with the following steps.

Step 1

First get on your knees with your palms on the floor so that your torso is parallel to the ground. To quickly visualize the starting position of this exercise, think of the starting position of a push-up with the only exception of your knees touching the floor.

Step 2

Then keep your left leg planted on the ground, and raise your right leg as high as you can. Then bring it back down till your knee is a few inches off the ground.

Step 3

Then do the same steps and the same number of reps and sets with your left leg.

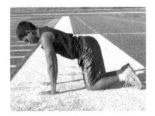 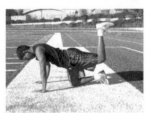 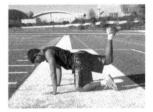

Tip 2.5: For novices, I recommend doing 5 to 10 reps for 5 sets. For the more advanced athletes, I suggest reps in the range of 15 to 25 for 4 to 6 sets.

Wall Chair

This exercise focuses on the quadriceps and uses other leg muscles as supporting muscles.

Step 1

First stand up straight.

Step 2

Lower yourself till you are at a 90-degree lock with your legs or the lowest position of a squat. This is the chair position.

Step 3

Stay in that chair position for the amount of time required.

When you do this exercise, make sure that your back is firmly planted against a wall, hence the name *wall chair*. If you are extremely fit, then you can do this exercise without a wall for support.

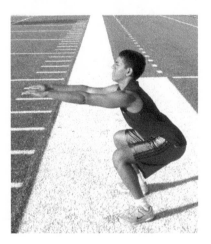

Tip 2.6: For novices, I suggest doing this exercise for 10 seconds for 3 to 5 sets. For the experienced, I recommend hitting 30 seconds to 1 minute for 3 to 5 sets.

Jumps

The last lower body exercise we will talk about before moving on to abdominal workouts is jumps.

Step 1

Stand up straight.

Step 2

Then go down to the lowest position of a squat.

Step 3

Jump straight up.

This is a great exercise for burning calories and toning your legs.

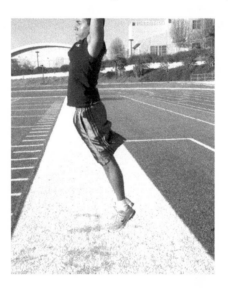

Tip 2.7: Put your hands up when you jump so that you have more stability. I also recommend that you do some jumps to get the form down. If you are a beginner, then I recommend between 5 and 10 reps for 3 sets. If you are in shape, then do 15 to 25 reps for 3 sets. If you really want to do work, then go beast mode by doing *30 plus reps for 3 sets!*

Abdominal Exercises

There are quite a few exercises for abdominals. But we will stick to the basics that give the best results. The first abdominal exercise I will go over is the classic sit-up.

Sit-ups

Sit-ups can become challenging because they use your abdominals continuously, rep after rep. I am sure that everyone who is reading this guide knows what a sit-up is. But for sanity's sake, let me explain how to do a proper sit-up.

Step 1

First lie down with your face and torso facing up, and make sure that your hands are at your sides.

Step 2

Then bend your legs so that your knees go up.

Step 3

Raise your upper body up till it is perpendicular to the ground.

Step 4

Slowly start to go back down to the starting position.

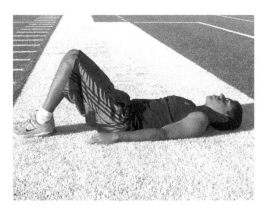

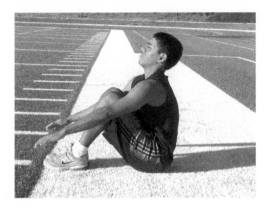

Tip 2.8: I recommend 3 sets of 5 to 10 reps for beginners, and 3 sets of 15 plus reps are recommended for experienced athletes.

Overhead Raise

The next abdominal exercise is what I call the overhead raise.

To do this exercise, follow these steps:

Step 1

First lie down with your face up and your hands on your sides or tucked underneath your butt. If you keep your hands on your sides, then the exercise will become much more challenging.

Step 2

Raise your legs straight up until they are perpendicular to the ground.

Step 3

Then slowly lower your legs till they are about a couple of inches off the ground.

Repeat these steps to complete other reps.

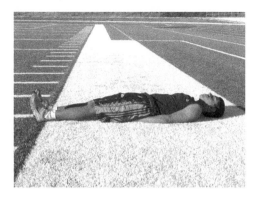

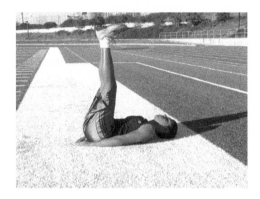

Tip 2.9: When raising and lowering your legs, make sure that they are as straight as a board. This exercise works your lower abdominals much more than your upper abs. For novices, I recommend 10 reps of 4 sets. If you go crazy and do 15 plus reps of 10 sets, expect your lower abs to get fatigued.

Scissors

Scissors are the most effective abdominal exercises that are time based. Follow these steps to perform scissors.

Step 1

First lie down with your face facing up and your hands underneath your buttocks or on your sides. The workout will be much more intense if you put your hands on your sides. This is the same concept I mentioned earlier with overhead raises.

Step 2

Raise both of your legs so that they are about a foot off the ground, and make sure that they are as straight as possible.

Step 3

Raise one leg up an additional distance of 6 to 12 inches from the starting position in step 2, then bring it back down.

Step 4

Then right when you bring that leg down to a foot off the ground, raise the other leg the same distance (6 to 12 inches).

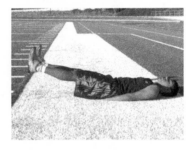

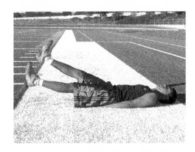

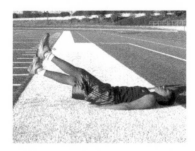

The switching of your legs should be in a continuous motion. You may need to practice getting your form down. So don't hesitate to work on your form! Once you master the form, then you will be ready to punish your abdominals set after set. Because you have to time yourself, you should have a stopwatch close by. You could even count the seconds in your head.

Tip 2.10: Novice athletes should perform this exercise for 5 to 10 seconds for 2 to 3 sets. Proficient athletes should perform this exercise for 30 seconds to 1 minute for 3 to 5 sets.

Planks

The next abdominal exercise is the plank. Planks are time based, and the form is really easy to master.

Step 1

First lie face down on the ground with your back facing up.

Step 2

Get into the push-up starting position.

Step 3

Have your forearms touch the ground. Your upper arms should be perpendicular to the ground, and your entire body should be as straight as a board.

Step 4

Stay in that position till the time for the set is finished.

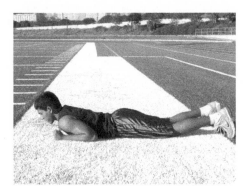

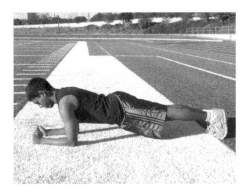

Tip 2.11: The novice athlete should go for 10 to 20 seconds for 2 to 4 sets. Proficient athletes should hit a time between 30 seconds and 1 minute for 3 to 5 sets.

Side Planks

Obliques are muscles on the sides of your abdominal wall. Side planks work the obliques and are harder to do than regular planks. They are time based.

Step 1

First get into the regular plank position.

Step 2

Turn your body sideways so that your right elbow is out.

Step 3

Make your body as straight as a plank, and stick your left arm straight up.

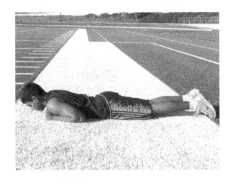

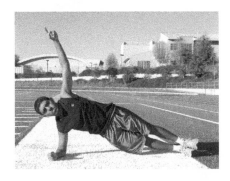

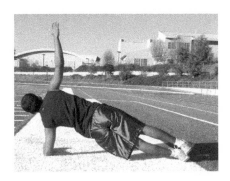

Tip 2.12: Novice athletes should perform this exercise for 5 to 15 seconds for 2 sets each side. Proficient athletes should aim for 20 seconds to 1 minute for 4 sets each side.

Now, on to the distance-running chapter!

CHAPTER 3

DISTANCE RUNNING

Just to keep it simple, consider distance running as just running a decent amount of mileage at a certain level of intensity. Competing in events may require help from a coach. There are a lot of respectable books written on distance running cited in the references section.

Distance running can be really fun, especially if you run with a friend. If you run with a friend on a scenic route, then you are likely to run more often. I personally believe that not only is long-distance running the easiest way to get into shape but also can be pleasurable and relieve stress from work or school. For example, let's say you are studying hard for a difficult test and getting stressed because the test is tomorrow. Then you say, "I'm going to take a break by going for a light run." You begin jogging and look at the beautiful sunset. After a good 20 minutes, you come home feeling stress free and relaxed, exactly what you need for next day.

Distance running is an established area of fitness. There are different types of training for distance running starting from amateur running to 5 kilometers, 10 kilometers, half marathon, full marathon, half ironman, and ironman to ultramarathons (25 kilometers or farther). There are special workout books to train for these distances (McGee, etc.). It is not the focus of this chapter to address these workouts, but I will give a couple of distance workouts. The key aspects of distance running are distance, route, and hydration.

The importance of mileage depends on what you want to achieve in your long-distance workouts. A distance of 2 to 3 miles at good intensity gets calories burned fast. A distance run where you want to hit 5 plus miles (approximately 8 kilometers), at a jogging pace, will burn calories slowly. But 5-plus-mile runs are for prodistance runners, not for amateurs who are trying to get in shape. If you are not training for a marathon and if you only want to get into shape, then 4 to 5 miles would be a good target.

The second aspect you should consider when running long distance is the route. Do you want to go through heavy intersections and urban roadways or run through beautiful suburbs that are clear of traffic or go on mountain roads? Long-distance running can become really enjoyable if you are on a clear road and have a fascinating view. Long-distance running can also be really enjoyable if you combine the scenic route with a bit of early morning sunshine in urban areas.

For example, consider my experience running a route around Hussain Sagar (*Sagar* in the Indian language of Hindi means "a water body like a natural lake, manmade reservoir, or even an ocean") in the heart of Hyderabad, India. I ran a full circle around the lake back in my ninth grade summer vacation. The route was about 7 miles long, and I had never run that distance before. It was sunrise when I ran; the sun produced sparkles in the water, which made the lake look beautiful. Since the Hussain Sagar route was free of smog, I enjoyed my run even more because the fresh air made the run relaxing. Now you may think that relaxation and distance running don't go together, but they actually do in certain conditions such as scenery, clean air, and the time of the day.

Finally, the last aspect of running is proper hydration in your long-distance running workouts! Distance running depletes you of your water weight, so you must make sure that you are well hydrated before you run. And also, you should make sure to sip some water with minerals like sodium, etc., here and there in your workouts. One should also cut down on caffeinated drinks like coffee before long runs.

Tip 3.1: You should be drinking water constantly throughout the day.

I will review precautions, stretching for distance running, and two sample workouts in this chapter.

Precautions

When Running in Hot Weather

Make sure you take precautions when you run in the heat. Running in boiling weather without precautions can be dangerous. When you run in the heat, your body has to work harder than it would in running at an ideal temperature.

1. Do your runs in the evening or early morning because the temperature is much cooler.
2. If the temperature is hot or rising, then do an easy workout. You will not be able to complete heavy workouts when the temperature is beyond the ideal temperature to run in, which is around 60 degrees Fahrenheit.
3. Try not to run between 10:00 a.m. and 4:00 p.m. so that you can prevent sunburns! Also when you run, make sure you put sunscreen with an SPF of at least 30.

When Running in Cold weather or Winter

1. Lessen your stride so that you won't slip and fall.
2. Keep an eye on where you are stepping. Freshly fallen snow can cover strips of ice.
3. Run during midday because most of the ice will melt, and it will be the warmest time of the day.
4. Suit up properly for the cold. You should have running gear that blocks the wind, and wear mittens or gloves.

Stretches

You should perform these stretches before and after your runs so that you don't pull a muscle or feel excessively sore the next day.

Quadriceps/Hip Flexor Stretch

1. Stand on your knees with your body facing straight.
2. Bring your right leg forward while keeping the left knee on the floor.
3. Keep your shoulders back, and push your hips forward.
4. Your knee on the leg placed forward should not extend past the front of your feet.
5. Hold this stretch for 25 to 30 seconds.
6. Then put your left leg forward, and repeat the process.

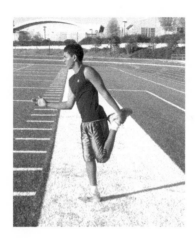

Standing Calf Raise

1. Stand straight.
2. Bring the heel of your left foot down while keeping the ball of the foot on the step or platform.
3. Keep your upper body as straight as possible.
4. Put your body weight on your left leg.
5. Keep your left knee as straight as possible in order to fully stretch the calf.
6. Hold the stretch for 25 to 30 seconds.
7. Repeat the process with your right calf.

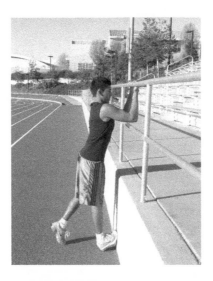

Distance-Running Workouts

If you want to do a simple long-distance workout just to burn some calories and get your heart pumping, then hit 5 miles on a level ground at a nice and easy pace. This may take a few weeks after a preconditioning phase where you are only able to cover 2 to 4 miles per run. Try to finish the 5 miles between 50 and 55 minutes. If your level of fitness is very good, then aim for 3 to 4 miles, and try to hit that mileage in 25 to 35 minutes.

Tip 3.2: If you want to increase the intensity of the workout, then I recommend adding in a mini-abdominal workout halfway through your run. The abdominal workout doesn't have to be too long; it should be in the range of 5 to 10 sets. Each set in the brief abdominal workout should be roughly around the intensity of 10 to 30 sit-ups.

If are still lost on what long-distance running workouts to try out, check out a couple of my favorite long-distance running workouts below:

Workout 1: Wolf Pack Run

Gather at least two to three friends to run with.

Step 1: Head over to a track-and-field track and warm up. It's going to be a tough workout, so get your game face on!

Step 2: Get in a straight line with all your friends.

Step 3: Go to the end of the line. Runner 1 is first in line, and you are last.

Step 4: When the run starts, everyone jogs in a single line around the track for the first lap.

Step 5: Immediately after the first lap, move into the right lane, and run to get to the front of the pack. Now you are the alpha wolf and line leader.

Step 6: As soon as you get to the front, the last person in the line will run to get to the front and will replace you. To keep it simple, one person runs on the side of the pack to get to the front of the line. When that person gets to the front of the line, the last person in line will repeat what the previous person did.

Step 7: Have the pack run in this formation for 8 laps on the track (about 2 miles total distance). Keep in mind the raw intensity of the workout. When I did this workout for the first time, it was so bad that immediately after finishing all 8 laps, I fell on the track and rested for 5 minutes.

Step 8: Cool down and stretch with your friends.

Step 9: Relax for the rest of the day or even take the next day off. You earned it.

Workout 2: The Morning Love

This is a morning workout that starts your day right.

Step 1: Get up before sunrise, and get ready to run. Bring a camera or iPhone if you want to take some beautiful pictures.

Step 2: Do your warm-up and stretches until sunrise.

Step 3: Start running wherever you are ready at medium intensity when sunrise starts.

Step 4: After 20 minutes of running, stop for a body-weight workout. For the workout below, have a rest interval of 45 to 60 seconds between sets.

- 5 sets of sit-ups for 15-20 reps
- 5 sets of overhead raises for 15-20 reps
- 3 sets of planks for 1 minute each
- 3 sets of push-ups for 15 reps
- 3 sets of tricep dips for 10 reps
- 3 sets of tricep push-ups for 15 reps

Step 5: Take 2 minutes' break after the body-weight workout.

Step 6: Start running again at medium intensity for 15 minutes.

Step 7: Cool down after the workout.

Now that we covered long-distance running, it's time to go to the next chapter on nutrition and rest!

CHAPTER 4

NUTRITION AND SLEEP

We have covered three areas of fitness in the first three chapters of this book. In this chapter and the next, we will examine other areas of health, including nutrition and sleep. These areas require only good habits but do not consume time, like the workouts previously discussed.

The saying "You are what you eat" is mostly correct. I will explain about the exception to this quote later, but for now, let's stick to why you should eat healthy and what and how much you should eat. I packed my lunch for school during track-and-field season since my school cafeteria's food choices did not provide a balanced diet.

So why should you eat healthy? Well, if you want to get into shape, eating a proper balance of proteins, carbohydrates, and fats will benefit you. Benefits include enhancing recovery process and providing essential nutrients. A nutritious diet is crucial because you need to be as fresh and healthy as you can be. You will be fresher throughout the day when you get the nutrients your body needs.

I will give you a basic overview of nutrition, including aspects that apply to athletes and finally about sleep and rest.

Nutrition Food Groups

Let us take a different approach to nutrition from the well-known food pyramid. Instead of taking x servings of vegetables and fruits, whole grains, dairy products, and meat and poultry, let us review the nutrition facts of food groups. You should be concerned about your protein, carbohydrate, fat, and fiber intake in your daily diet. Protein is used to repair your muscles; therefore, it is vital to take in foods that are high in protein, such as skinless chicken breasts, nuts, and lentils. A rule of thumb for people who exercise and want to get into shape is to consume 0.8 grams of protein for every pound of body weight. If you are large and have trouble getting your daily amount of protein, then buy protein powder and drink protein shakes. There are about 20 to 30 grams of protein on average in a protein shake. That's a lot of protein!

Carbohydrates are vital for energy. The more carbohydrates you take in, the more energy you will have, which means performing better in workouts. What about the simple-carbs-versus-complex-carbs debate? Simple carbs are very low in nutritional value and are very easy to digest. You should limit your consumption of simple carbs. Simple carbohydrates are refined sugars that can be found in foods such as white rice, candy, cake, soda, packaged cereals, and products made with white flour. Complex carbohydrates are sugars that are rich in minerals, fiber, and vitamins. Complex carbs also contribute greatly to energy production by acting as your body's fuel. Complex carbs can be found in foods such as broccoli, spinach, yams, beans, and whole-grain breads.

Next, it is important to be knowledgeable about fats because they don't necessarily make you gain weight. You gain weight by eating in excess. For example, let's say you eat 500 calories in excess every day of the week. This totals out to a weekly excess of 3,500 calories, which is equal to 1 pound of fat. So every week, you would gain about 1 pound of fat.

Good fats should be about 20% of your daily calorie intake. Good fats are polyunsaturated fats, monounsaturated fats, and omega-3s. Good fats are in foods like peanuts, almonds, avocados, walnuts, and fish like salmon, trout, and tuna. However, don't eat 20% of bad fat! Bad fats are trans fats and saturated fats. Trans fats are in processed food, some frozen food, chips, crackers, and candy. Saturated fats are in dairy, meat, and deep-fried foods.

What about fiber? Fiber is part of all vegetables and fruits and whole grains in addition to vitamins and minerals. There are two types of fiber: soluble and insoluble. Soluble fiber is soluble in water and is absorbed into blood, and insoluble fiber doesn't dissolve in water and cleans your digestive track. A high-fiber diet gives benefits such as lowering cholesterol levels, achieving a healthy weight, and controlling blood sugar levels, and even improving joint strength. Men and women fifty years old or younger need 38 grams and 25 grams per day respectively. Men and women over fifty years old need 30 grams and 21 grams per day respectively.

Now that we talked about balanced nutrition, do you ever wonder if one could indulge in fast food or desserts occasionally? The answer is yes, and athletes call them cheat meals, but they are very disciplined about the frequency and timing of consuming these meals. For the most part, they eat a well-balanced diet.

Athletes' Nutrition

Many athletes have cheat meals when they are in season (time of year when competing). Athletes can't afford to eat junk food in season, so they have cheat meals and, for some, cheat days. A cheat meal is a meal that is usually eaten weekly to biweekly. It is a meal you eat that contains whatever junk food you've craved for in the past week or two. If athletes consume healthy food consistently, then they would eventually succumb to junk food because over time, the desire to eat junk builds stronger. I wouldn't be surprised if some athletes go to the closet at night and cry while munching on some delicious chocolate-glazed donuts. If you want to get into good shape, then I advise you to have one to two cheat meals a week. There are also cheat days for food. A cheat day is when you eat junk food for more than one meal in a day. Not many people have cheat days.

Some people may ask why some athletes eat junk food all the time but are still very high up in their respective sports. The answer to this question is that in some sports, at certain phases, you need to consume so many calories that eating junk food doesn't make a difference. These athletes get to a stage in their sports where they eat heaps of junk food to get easy calories in. To them, junk food no longer acts as junk food; it acts as food that has many calories and is easier to eat than piles of healthy food.

One example of someone eating a calorie surplus of junk food is my friend who is on the swim team at his high school. He is one of the best swimmers at his school and eats everything in his path. He told me he ate pizza almost every day and other foods that were mostly junk. He was only eating like this in off-season (time of year when athletes train heavily to better themselves). Eating 3,000 calories every day off-season helps him progress in his sport because it gives him the energy to train intensely for 2 to 3 hours a day.

The main side effect of eating in excess for an athlete is gaining unwanted weight, usually in the form of pure fat. However, my friend is not concerned about packing on flab because it helps him float easily in water. Having the ability to float easily when you are a competitive swimmer is a significant advantage.

Another example of calorie-excess eating is my friend who is a competitive bodybuilder. In bulking season (time period where bodybuilders pack on muscle mass), he eats 1,000 excess calories daily. The calorie excess helps him increase his muscle mass as well as some fat. Since bodybuilders' primary focus in bulking season is packing on muscle mass, the extra pounds of flab don't concern them.

This sums up the topic of eating excess food for certain sports or for certain phases of sports. Remember, what I talked on about cheat meals and junk food will most likely not concern you if you want to get into shape and be fit, so don't worry about calorie excesses. Just focus on eating healthy in the proper proportions, and have a cheat meal once in a while. Also use a BMR calculator online (http://exrx.net/Calculators/CalRequire.html) to see how much calorie intake you need daily.

Before I end this chapter, I need to talk about sleep/rest since it is the key to good energy levels and recovery after workouts.

Sleep

Sleep is the most important factor of rest. Did you know that fifty to seventy million people in the USA live on the edge of mental/physical collapse because they lack proper sleep? The statistics are shocking. Let me explain why a good night's sleep is important, the science of sleep, causes and cures of insomnia, and some pointers for getting better sleep so that you can have proper workouts and recovery.

Lack of sleep is detrimental to your health. When you sleep less, say five to six hours a day, your body can't rejuvenate in time for the next day. Many people boast that they sleep little and can still perform functions reasonably well. However, they take energy pills or energy drinks to keep themselves up. Consuming those pills and drinks isn't good for you.

During the hours you sleep, your body goes into a relaxed state and repairs itself for the grueling tasks of tomorrow. When you sleep, you release important hormones, such as growth hormone and leptin. Growth hormone regulates growth in children, helps watch fat levels in adults, and manages muscle mass. Leptin influences your appetite by telling you when your stomach is full. If you don't have enough leptin, then you tend to eat in excess, which will lead to negative weight gain.

What are the benefits of getting good sleep? The most important benefit is improvement of your brain function. This means that you perform tasks at a higher level and become more alert. Don't you want to feel alive during the day? Sleep is your solution!

Sleeping well for the right amount of time can decelerate the aging process. The right amount of sleep should be between seven and nine hours for most people. How long you will live can easily be predicted by how well and how much you sleep. Evidence shows that by having deficient sleep, your life span can shorten by eight to ten years. You want to live longer and age more slowly, right? Then sleep well for the right amount of time! Check to see if you are getting quality sleep for seven to nine hours from today.

Another benefit of sleep is that it reduces cortisol levels, which play havoc with the neurotransmitter balance in the brain. The result is, you are more prone to apprehension, depression, and insomnia. Insomnia is an extremely common sleep disorder. People with insomnia have trouble falling asleep or staying asleep and, in worst cases, have trouble with both.

Insomniacs require knowledge of the sleep stages, reasons for having troubled sleep, and cures for troubled sleep in order to sleep well. So let us first understand the science of the sleep process.

Sleep happens in cycles, with each cycle lasting between sixty and ninety minutes. Majority of people complete about five to six cycles in the duration of their sleep. Each cycle has two parts. The first part is made up of four stages. People's bodies get the most rest in the third and fourth stages. The second part of sleep cycles involves rapid eye movement (REM), which is more commonly known as REM sleep. This is where dreams occur. People spend few minutes in the REM sleep in the first cycle; however, after each cycle, more time is spent in the REM sleep. REM sleep becomes the majority of people's last sleep cycle when they wake up. If you wake up in REM sleep, then you will remember your dreams more clearly.

Many insomniacs are unaware of the reasons for their troubled sleep. Many people can't get a good night's rest because of stress and apprehension, caffeine, cigarettes and alcohol, exercise, terrible pillow or mattress, and environment or background.

Stress and apprehension are the main causes of insomnia. People lie on their beds pondering about problems and important events that will happen the next day or in the distant future. People also try to think about fixing issues that cause them worry, such as relationships. Folks do all this in bed because it is so easy to have thoughts zooming through their minds when lying down. The cure for this cause of insomnia is to have a journal and write in it for twenty minutes before you sleep. Put all your thoughts in the journal, and I mean *everything*. Worried that your girlfriend is going to break up with you? Then write about it in your journal. By doing this, you are emptying out your mind before you go to bed. Once you finish writing in your journal and go to bed, say to yourself, "I don't have to think about anything. It's time to relax. I deserve this."

Tip 4.1: Another cure for stress is to do meditation for 20 minutes once or twice every day.

Tip 4.2: Don't exercise within three hours before sleeping. If you do, then your stress hormone levels will rise, which could *potentially* interfere with your sleep.

Many people drink liquids that have caffeine, such as iced teas, coffee, and sodas. Caffeine can stay in your body for up to twenty hours. That's a long time! Many people can't sleep because they drink caffeine. Caffeine shortens the amount of sleep you get because it makes you alert and keeps you awake much longer.

Tip 4.3: Limit your caffeinated drink to one or two cups a day before noon.

Cigarettes and alcohol hinder you from getting a good night's rest. People believe by drinking alcohol, they will be able to fall asleep easily and will sleep well. However, this is not true because alcohol interferes with sleep stages. Therefore, they sleep light and would wake up the next day feeling groggy or sluggish. Nicotine, a chemical from cigarettes, releases adrenaline in the body, which often leads to insomnia. So don't smoke or drink alcohol!

An obvious cause of insomnia is having a terrible pillow or uncomfortable mattress. Invest in a good pillow and mattress with the firmness that suits you. You may be unwilling to spend a considerable amount of money on a mattress or pillow, so think about this situation. You are going to be spending time on your bed for seven to nine hours a day, which is about a third of your day. Since you will be spending so much time on a bed, then why not invest in a comfortable mattress and pillow?

The background and environment you sleep in can cause insomnia. You need to be able to sleep in your room, so you have to make it perfect for sleeping. The prime purpose of your bedroom is for sleeping. According to a National Sleep Foundation poll, 40% of Americans reported having computer (laptops, desktops, or tablets) in their bedroom and 3% would even leave the light on all night in their bedroom. Exposure to light during sleep reduces the sleep hormone, melatonin, according to a Rensselaer Polytechnic Institute study.

Last but not the least, your bedroom should not be a storage unit. When people go into bedrooms to sleep and there are items all over the place, then their minds get confused. The mind sees the room as a place to be productive and busy. So empty your room out. The computer, television set, and articles should all go into a room where you are not sleeping. Make sure your room doesn't have light coming in from your bedroom windows (put shades, etc.).

Tip 4.4: One practical tip you can follow when you are trying to sleep better is to have a sleeping journal for two weeks. It is important to keep a two-week journal titled "My Sleep" so that you can analyze why you didn't get a good night's snooze for a certain day based on collected evidence. A sample journal is included below:

Week 1

Day of the Week	How do I feel about my sleep? Ex: Good, wasn't good, okay, bad till midnight	Number of hours I slept Goal: seven to nine hours	Time I went to bed and got out of bed	Things I did in my sleep time that I should stop for a better night's sleep
Sunday				
Monday				
Tuesday				
Wednesday				
Thursday				
Friday				
Saturday				

Week 2

Day of the Week	How do I feel about my sleep? Ex: Good, wasn't good, okay, bad till midnight	Number of hours I slept Goal: seven to nine hours	Time I went to bed and got out of bed	Things I did in my sleep time that I should stop for a better night's sleep
Sunday				
Monday				
Tuesday				
Wednesday				
Thursday				
Friday				
Saturday				

Tip 4.5: Take a short nap (say 20 minutes) in the afternoon if possible. Naps recharge you, increase alertness for the rest of the day, and increase your capacity to complete tasks.

Armed with the knowledge of nutrition and sleep from this chapter and different exercise workouts from the earlier chapters, let us move on to the next chapter for sample two-week nutrition and workout plans for beginner, intermediate, and advanced levels of fitness.

CHAPTER 5

NUTRITION AND WORKOUT PLANS

Knowledge of health and fitness is not useful unless there is goal setting and preparation and execution of good plans. These actions and habits provide expected results. I made an attempt to provide sample two-week nutrition and workout plans in this chapter. By all means, you can formulate your own plans, but make sure you execute them. You will start seeing results in as little as a few weeks!

Sample nutrition and workout plans are organized as beginner, intermediate, and advanced levels. For each of these levels, there are two-week plans for sprinting, distance running, and body-weight training. There is also a two-week cross-training plan for beginner level, combining sprinting, distance running, and strength training. It may take up to six to eight weeks to graduate from each level. Once you reach advanced level, keep pushing your body with more challenging cross-training and even adding machines.

For nutrition, I recommend fresh food choices like fish, eggs, poultry, fruits, vegetables, nuts and grains, etc. Prepare meals at home as much as you can. The nutrition plans in this chapter use meals that anyone can prepare at home. If you are looking for recipes, there are many recipe books out there. The one I like is *The Skinny Rules* by Bob Harper.

General guidelines for calorie intake depend on age; gender; beginner, intermediate, or advanced level workouts; body weight; and BMI number. The range is from 1,200 to 2,000 calories per day.

Some general nutritional tips are included below.

Tip 5.1: Drink water throughout the day (no liquid calories—I mean soda or juices), and drink a glass of water before every meal.

Tip 5.2: Add berries to your cereal or oatmeal for taste.

Tip 5.3: Try to include one apple and some berries every day in your diet.

Tip 5.4: Add a plateful of steamed vegetables (or two) if you do not feel full with main meals, but I recommend eating a bowl of green salad with fat-free dressing as first course for dinner (if you have time to prepare).

Tip 5.5: If you like fish, you can substitute fish (preferably wild-caught fish) for steak and poultry in these plans.

Tip 5.6: Choose whole grain or multigrain flour or bread to meet fiber requirements instead of refined flours or white bread.

Tip 5.7: Include yams and bananas in your diet for high potassium levels to help with muscle recovery on hard exercise days.

Tip 5.8: Have plenty of citrus fruits in your daily diet to increase vitamin C levels. Advanced level workouts may need a vitamin C supplement, but consult your physician or nutritionist before taking any vitamin supplements.

Tip 5.9: Eat a low-fat dessert with dinner on hard exercise days, but limit portion size. You earned it!

Tip 5.10: Eat an ounce of nuts or a cup of low-fat fruit yogurt as a bedtime snack if your dinnertime and bedtime are spaced about three hours so that you do not get up in the middle of night craving for food because of low blood glucose levels!

Tip 5.11: You should eat no earlier than two hours before your workout, and the optimal time to work out is *between* 2:00 p.m. and 6:00 p.m.

Tip 5.12: Avoid fast foods (except maybe cheat meals discussed in the last chapter) and packaged processed foods at all cost, including frozen dinners.

Two-Week Plan, Sprinting: Beginner Level

Day	Nutrition Plan	Workout Plan
Sunday	Breakfast: 3-egg-white omelet with two slices of whole multigrain bread and fat-free milk Snack 1: fistful of almonds with milk Lunch: pasta and grilled chicken and 2 cups of vegetables Snack 2: 1 apple and 4-12 berries Dinner: brown rice and 2 cups (each is 1 to 1.5 of FDA servings) of vegetables	5 × 100 meter sprints 75% top speed Rest interval: 1 minute between sprints
Monday	Breakfast: two to four 1-oz. to 1.5-oz. packets of oatmeal with milk Snack 1: milk and 1 banana Lunch: turkey-and-cheese sandwich with 2 slices of multigrain bread with pasta-sauce spread Snack 2: milk with a serving of mixed nuts Dinner: pasta with fish, 2 cups of broccoli, and an apple	Rest day! You are a beginner, so you will need extra recovery time from your first day of training!
Tuesday	Breakfast: 2 cups of cereal with milk Snack 1: milk and 2 cups of fruits Lunch: brown rice, vegetables, and chicken Snack 2: fistful of almonds and milk Dinner: fast food of your choice (Big Macs or chalupas)	1 lap of UCLAs

Wednesday	Breakfast: 2-egg-white omelet with orange juice Snack 1: 2 cups of fruits with milk Lunch: turkey and cream cheese bagel Snack 2: 2 cups of vegetables with apple juice Dinner: pasta and turkey meatballs	4 × 50 meter sprints uphill All-out top speed Go hard or go home!
Thursday	Breakfast: 2-egg-white omelet with 2 slices of bread and milk Snack 1: 1 apple Lunch: pasta and grilled chicken Snack 2: 1 orange Dinner: brown rice with fish and 1 cup of vegetables	Rest day! Your body still needs to adapt to working out.
Friday	Breakfast: 2 to 4 packets of oatmeal with milk Snack 1: 2 cups of fruits Lunch: peanut butter sandwich Snack 2: 2 cups of vegetables with milk Dinner: noodles and steak	2 × 600 meter sprints 70% top speed Rest interval: 4 minutes
Saturday	Breakfast: 3 packets of oatmeal with milk Snack 1: 2 cups of vegetables Lunch: peanut butter sandwich Snack 2: milk and a slice of bread spread with almond butter Dinner: noodles with fish and 2 cups of fruits	Rest day!

Sunday	Breakfast: 2 cups of cereal with milk Snack 1: milk and 2 cups of vegetables Lunch: brown rice and steak Snack 2: 2 cups of fruits and milk Dinner: Fish fillet and peanut butter sandwich	2 × 50 meter sprints and 2 × 100 meter sprints 80% top speed
Monday	Breakfast: 1 cup of cereal and 1 slice of french toast Snack 1: milk and 2 cups of fruits Lunch: peanut butter sandwich and 2 cups of vegetables Snack 2: handful of mixed nuts Dinner: pasta with fish and 2 cups of vegetables	4 × 400 meter sprints 80% top speed
Tuesday	Breakfast: 2 slices of french toast with milk Snack 1: milk and 2 cups of fruits Lunch: steak meatballs and pasta Snack 2: 3 cups of vegetables Dinner: turkey-and-cheese sandwich	Rest day!
Wednesday	Breakfast: 2 cups of cereal with milk Snack 1: milk and 2 cups of vegetables Lunch: ham-and-cheese sandwich Snack 2: handful of peanuts Dinner: pasta with fish and 2 cups of vegetables	4 sets of accelerations

Thursday	Breakfast: 2-egg-white omelet with juice Snack 1: milk and cookies Lunch: brown rice with 2 cups of vegetables Snack 2: 3 cups of fruits Dinner: 1 Big Mac or eat what you are craving at the moment!	Rest day!
Friday	Breakfast: 3 packets of oatmeal with milk Snack 1: 3 cups of fruits Lunch: peanut butter sandwich Snack 2: milk and a slice of bread spread with jelly Dinner: noodles and grilled chicken and 2 cups of vegetables	4 × 200 meter sprints Rest interval: 2 minutes 80% top speed
Saturday	Breakfast: 2-egg omelet with a slice of bread Snack 1: milk and a slice of bread spread with jelly Lunch: ham-and-cheese sandwich Snack 2: 3 cups of fruits Dinner: noodles and steak and 3 cups of vegetables	Rest day!

Two-Week Plan Sprinting: Intermediate Level

Day	Nutrition Plan	Workout Plan
Sunday	Breakfast: peanut butter and jelly sandwich and milk Snack 1: 3 cups of fruits Lunch: turkey-and-cheese sandwiches Snack 2: a handful of mixed nuts Dinner: brown rice with fish and 4 cups of vegetables	6 × 200 meter sprints Rest interval: 2 minutes 85-90% top speed
Monday	Breakfast: 3 cups of cereal with milk Snack 1: 4 cups of vegetables Lunch: brown rice and grilled chicken Snack 2: 3 cups of fruits Dinner: 2 slices of homemade pizza	2 laps (sets) of UCLAs 80% top speed Rest interval: 5 minutes
Tuesday	Breakfast: 1-large-egg omelet with milk Snack 1: 2 mangos or other large fruits Lunch: noodles and grilled chicken Snack 2: 4 cups of vegetables Dinner: brown rice and fish	5 × 400 meter sprints Rest interval: 5 minutes 85% top speed
Wednesday	Breakfast: 3-small-egg omelet with milk Snack 1: 3 peaches Lunch: white rice and steak Snack 2: 2 oranges Dinner: 2 homemade chicken and rice burritos	Rest day!

Thursday	Breakfast: 4 packets of oatmeal with milk Snack 1: 2 apples Lunch: brown rice, fish, and 1 cup of vegetables Snack: 2 bananas Dinner: turkey-and-cheese sandwiches	4 × 600 meter sprints 90% top speed Rest interval: 4 minutes
Friday	Breakfast: 3 cups of cereal with milk Snack 1: 2 mangos Lunch: fast food of your choice Snack 2: 1 banana Dinner: chicken and rice burritos	6 × 100 meter sprints Rest interval: 90 seconds 85% top speed
Saturday	Breakfast: 2 cups of cereal with milk Snack 1: 3 cups of fruits Lunch: ham-and-cheese sandwiches Snack 2: 3 cups of vegetables Dinner: multigrain pasta with fish	Rest day!
Sunday	Breakfast: 2 cups of cereal with milk Snack 1: 2 cups of fruits Lunch: ham-and-cheese sandwiches Snack 2: handful of peanuts Dinner: brown rice, fish, and 2 cups of vegetables	7 × 50 meter uphill sprints All out Rest interval: 2 minutes
Monday	Breakfast: 2-large-egg omelet and milk Snack 1: 3 cups of grapes Lunch: grain of your choice and 2 cups of vegetables Snack 2: fistful of mixed nuts Dinner: brown rice and grilled chicken	7 × 150 meter flat-ground sprints 90% top speed Rest interval: 2 to 3 minutes

Tuesday	Breakfast: 3 slices of french toast and milk Snack 1: 3 cups of vegetables Lunch: ham-and-cheese sandwiches Snack 2: 4 cups of fruits Dinner: multigrain pasta with fish, 2 cups of vegetables	Do the 400- and 200-meter relays with your friends Run a 400-meter leg and a 200-meter leg All-out top speed
Wednesday	Breakfast: 1-egg-omelet with 2 slices of turkey bacon Snack 1: 2 apples Lunch: turkey-and-bacon sandwich Snack 2: 3 cups of cherries Dinner: brown rice and steak	Rest day!
Thursday	Breakfast: fast food of your choice Snack 1: milk and 3 cups of fruits Lunch: 1-large-egg omelet with brown rice Snack 2: 4 cups of vegetables Dinner: steak and brown rice burritos	2 laps (sets) of UCLAs 85% top speed Rest interval: 5 minutes
Friday	Breakfast: 4 packets of oatmeal with milk Snack 1: milk and cookies Lunch: 1-large-egg omelet with brown rice Snack 2: 4 cups of vegetables Dinner: multigrain pasta with fish and 3 cups of fruits	6 × 50 meter flat-ground sprints 90% top speed Rest interval: 2 to 3 minutes
Saturday	Breakfast: 3 cups of cereal Snack 1: 3 cups of cherries/berries Lunch: turkey-and-cheese sandwiches Snack 2: milk and 3 cups of fruits Dinner: brown rice and steak and 2 cups of vegetables	Rest day!

Two-Week Plan, Sprinting: Advanced Level

Day	Nutrition Plan	Workout Plan
Sunday	Breakfast: 3-medium-egg omelet and milk Snack 1: 2 medium-sized bananas Lunch: ham-and-cheese sandwiches Snack 2: yogurt and 4 cups of watermelon Dinner: brown rice, fish and vegetables	2 sets of pyramid sprinting 90% top speed Rest interval: 5 minutes
Monday	Breakfast: 4 slices of french toast and milk Snack 1: 2 apples Lunch: white rice and steak, 3 cups vegetables Snack 2: yogurt and 3 cups of fruit Dinner: brown rice and grilled chicken and 3 cups of vegetables	3 laps (sets) of UCLAs 90% top speed Rest interval: 4 minutes
Tuesday	Breakfast: 3 cups of cereal with milk Snack 1: yogurt and 3 cups of fruits Lunch: chicken and rice burritos, 3 cups of vegetables Snack 2: 3 small bananas Dinner: fast food of your choice	5 × 400 meter sprints 90% top speed Rest interval: 5 minutes
Wednesday	Breakfast: 4 packets of oatmeal with milk Snack 1: yogurt and 1 cup of vegetables Lunch: peanut butter and jelly sandwich Snack 2: 2 cups of fruits Dinner: noodles and grilled chicken, 3 cups of vegetables	Rest day! Enjoy it!

Thursday	Breakfast: 4-small-egg omelet and milk Snack 1: 3 cups of vegetables Lunch: turkey-and-cheese sandwiches Snack 2: 3 cups of fruits Dinner: brown rice, fish, and 3 cups of vegetables	4 sets of accelerations Rest interval: 3 minutes
Friday	Breakfast: 3 cups of cereal with milk Snack 1: yogurt and 3 cups of vegetables Lunch: ham-and-cheese sandwiches Snack 2: 3 cups of fruits Dinner: pasta, fish, and 3 cups of vegetables	6 × 100 meter sprints 95% top speed Rest interval: 2 minutes
Saturday	Breakfast: 3-large-egg omelet and milk Snack 1: 4 cups of fruits Lunch: turkey-and-cheese sandwiches Snack 2: 4 cups of vegetables Dinner: brown rice and grilled chicken and 3 cups of vegetables	7 × 50 meter uphill sprints All-out top speed Rest interval: 4 minutes
Sunday	Breakfast: 5 slices of french toast and milk Snack 1: a handful of nuts and 2 cups of fruits Lunch: brown rice and 2 cups of vegetables Snack 2: 2 cups of fruits Dinner: chicken and rice burritos and 4 cups of vegetables	7 × 150 meter flat-ground sprints 95% top speed Rest interval: 4 minutes

Monday	Breakfast: 5 packets of oatmeal with milk Snack 1: 4 medium bananas or 3 cups of mixed fruits Lunch: chicken and brown rice burritos Snack 2: 4 cups of vegetables Dinner: brown rice and steak and 3 cups of vegetables	4 sets of accelerations Rest interval: 4 minutes
Tuesday	Breakfast: 4-small-egg omelet and milk Snack 1: milk and 1 cup of vegetables Lunch: peanut butter sandwiches Snack 2: 4 cups of fruits Dinner: brown rice, fish, and 4 cups of vegetables	6×200 meter sprints 95% top speed Rest interval: 3 minutes
Wednesday	Breakfast: 5 slices of french toast and milk Snack 1: 4 cups of vegetables Lunch: turkey-and-cheese sandwiches Snack 2: 4 cups of fruits and milk Dinner: brown rice and grilled chicken and 2 cups of vegetables	Rest day! You worked hard yesterday, so enjoy your rest day!
Thursday	Breakfast: 5 cups of cereal with milk Snack 1: 4 medium-sized bananas Lunch: chicken burritos and 2 cups of vegetables Snack 2: milk and cookies Dinner: noodles and fish and 3 cups of vegetables	3 laps (sets) of UCLAs 90% top speed Rest interval: 4 minutes

Friday	Breakfast: 5-small-egg omelet and milk Snack 1: 4 cups of fruits Lunch: ham-and-cheese sandwiches Snack 2: 4 cups of vegetables Dinner: fast food of your choice	7 × 600 meter sprints 90% top speed Rest interval: 5 minutes
Saturday	Breakfast: 5 slices of french toast and milk Snack 1: 4 cups of fruits and yogurt Lunch: brown rice and steak with 2 cups of vegetables Snack 2: 4 cups of fruits Dinner: chicken and rice burritos, 3 cups of vegetables	4 × 50 meter sprints and 4 × 100 meter sprints 90% top speed Rest interval between each sprint: 3 minutes

Two-Week Plan, Strength Training
(Body-Weight Exercises): Beginner Level

Day	Nutrition Plan	Workout Plan
Sunday	Breakfast: 3 slices of french toast and milk Snack 1: 2 cups of fruits and yogurt Lunch: chicken and rice burritos and 3 cups of vegetables Snack 2: handful of mixed nuts Dinner: brown rice, fish, and 3 cups of vegetables	Upper body day: 3 sets of push-ups, 5-10 reps 3 sets of tricep push-ups, 5-10 reps 3 sets of tricep dips, 5-10 reps Rest interval between sets: 30 seconds
Monday	Breakfast: 3 cups of cereal with milk Snack 1: 3 cups of vegetables Lunch: turkey-and-cheese sandwich Snack 2: 2 cups of fruits Dinner: noodles and steak and 3 cups of vegetables	Lower body day: 2 sets of squats, 5-15 reps 3 sets of glute-ups, 5-15 reps 3 sets of wall chair, 10-20 seconds 3 sets of jumps, 5 reps Rest interval between sets: 40 seconds
Tuesday	Breakfast: 3-small-egg omelet and milk Snack 1: 2 cups of fruits Lunch: ham-and-cheese sandwich Snack 2: yogurt and mixed nuts Dinner: brown rice, fish, and 2 cups of vegetables	Rest day!

Wednesday	Breakfast: 3 packets of oatmeal with milk Snack 1: milk and cookies Lunch: white rice and 2 cups of vegetables Snack 2: 2 cups of watermelon Dinner: chicken and rice burritos, 3 cups of vegetables	Abdominal day: 3 sets of sit-ups, 5-10 reps 3 sets of scissors, 10-20 seconds 3 sets of overhead raises, 5-15 reps Rest interval between sets: 40 seconds
Thursday	Breakfast: 3-small-egg omelet and milk Snack 1: fistful of walnuts Lunch: brown rice and 2 cups of vegetables Snack 2: 2 cups of watermelon Dinner: homemade pizza and 3 cups of vegetables (with yams)	Lower body day: 3 sets of jumps, 5 reps 2 sets of squats, 5-15 reps 3 sets of glute-ups, 5-15 reps 2 sets of wall chair, 10-20 seconds
Friday	Breakfast: 3 slices of french toast and milk Snack 1: 2 cups of vegetables Lunch: peanut butter sandwich and 3 cups of vegetables Snack 2: 2 apples Dinner: brown rice with fish and 3 cups of vegetables	Rest day!
Saturday	Breakfast: 3 slices of french toast and milk Snack 1: 2 cups of vegetables Lunch: fast food of your choice Snack 2: 2 cups of fruits and yogurt Dinner: brown rice with grilled chicken and 3 cups of vegetables	Rest day!

Sunday	Breakfast: 2-egg omelet and milk Snack 1: 2 cups of fruits Lunch: chicken and rice burritos and 3 cups of vegetables Snack 2: milk and a handful of cashews Dinner: brown rice with fish and 2 cups of vegetables	Upper body day: 3 sets of tricep dips, 5-10 reps 3 sets of tricep push-ups, 5-10 reps 3 sets of push-ups, 5-10 reps Rest interval between sets: 30 seconds
Monday	Breakfast: 3 cups of cereal with milk Snack 1: 2 cups of vegetables Lunch: ham-and-cheese sandwich, 2 cups of vegetables Snack 2: 2 cups of fruits and yogurt Dinner: noodles and grilled chicken, 3 cups of vegetables	Abdominal day: 3 sets of sit-ups, 5-10 reps 3 sets of scissors, 10-20 seconds 3 sets of overhead raises, 5-15 reps Rest interval between sets: 40 seconds
Tuesday	Breakfast: 3 packets of oatmeal with milk Snack 1: 2 cups of fruits and 2 cups of vegetables Lunch: 2-small-egg omelet with brown rice Snack 2: milk and cookies Dinner: pasta with fish, 3 cups of vegetables	Rest day!

Wednesday	Breakfast: 3-small-egg omelet with milk Snack 1: 2 cups of fruits Lunch: pasta with fish Snack 2: 2 cups of vegetables and yogurt Dinner: chicken and rice burritos, 3 cups of vegetables	Leg day: 2 sets of squats, 5-15 reps 3 sets of glute-ups, 5-15 reps 2 sets of wall chair, 10-20 seconds 3 sets of jumps, 5 reps Rest interval between sets: 40 seconds
Thursday	Breakfast: 3 packets of oatmeal with milk Snack 1: 2 cups of fruits Lunch: peanut butter and jelly sandwich Snack 2: 2 cups of vegetables Dinner: pasta and grilled chicken, 3 cups of vegetables	Upper body day: 3 sets of tricep push-ups, 5-10 reps 3 sets of tricep dips, 5-10 reps 3 sets of push-ups, 5-10 reps Rest interval between sets: 30 seconds
Friday	Breakfast: 3-egg-white omelet and milk Snack 1: 3 cups of fruits Lunch: turkey-and-cheese sandwich and 3 cups of vegetables Snack 2: 2 cups of vegetables and yogurt Dinner: brown rice with fish and 3 cups of vegetables	Rest day!
Saturday	Breakfast: 3 slices of french toast and milk Snack 1: 2 oranges/apples Lunch: noodles and steak Snack 2: 2 cups of vegetables and yogurt Dinner: fast food of your choice	Rest day!

Two-Week Plan, Strength Training
(Body-Weight Exercises): Intermediate Level

Day	Nutrition Plan	Workout Plan
Sunday	Breakfast: 4-small-egg omelet and orange juice Snack 1: 3 cups of vegetables and milk Lunch: turkey-and-cheese sandwiches and 3 cups of vegetables Snack 2: 3 cups of fruits and yogurt Dinner: brown rice, fish, and 3 cups of vegetables	Upper body day: 6 sets of push-ups, 10-20 reps 6 sets of tricep push-ups, 10-20 reps 6 sets of tricep dips, 10-20 reps Rest interval: 45 seconds to a minute
Monday	Breakfast: 5 slices of french toast and milk Snack 1: 3 cups of fruits Lunch: pasta and grilled chicken and 2 cups of vegetables Snack 2: 2 cups of vegetables and yogurt Dinner: pasta and steak and 2 cups of vegetables	Leg day: 5 sets of squats, 15-25 reps 5 sets of glute-ups, 20-25 reps 5 sets of wall chair, 30 seconds 5 sets of jumps, 8-10 reps Rest interval: 1 minute
Tuesday	Breakfast: 4 cups of cereal with milk Snack 1: fistful of cashews and 2 cups of vegetables Lunch: ham-and-cheese sandwiches Snack 2: 3 cups of fruits (preferably bananas) Dinner: pasta and fish, 3 cups of vegetables	Rest day!

Wednesday	Breakfast: 3-small-egg omelet and milk Snack 1: 3 cups of fruits Lunch: brown rice and 2 cups of broccoli Snack 2: yogurt and one cup of vegetables Dinner: noodles and steak, 3 cups of vegetables	Upper body day: 7 sets of tricep push-ups, 10-20 reps 7 sets of tricep dips, 10-20 reps 5 sets of push-ups, 10-20 reps Rest interval: 45 seconds to a minute
Thursday	Breakfast: 5 cups of cereal with milk Snack 1: 3 cups of fruits Lunch: noodles and 4 cups of vegetables Snack 2: handful of mixed nuts and yogurt Dinner: fast food of your choice!	Abdominal day: 5 sets of scissors, 30 seconds 5 sets of sit-ups, 10-25 reps 5 sets of overhead raises, 15-20 reps Rest interval: 40 seconds
Friday	Breakfast: 4 packets of oatmeal with milk Snack 1: 3 cups of vegetables Lunch: noodles and grilled chicken Snack 2: 3 cups of fruit salad and yogurt Dinner: brown rice and fish, 3 cups of vegetables	Rest day! Go do something fun!
Saturday	Breakfast: 4-medium-egg omelet and milk Snack 1: 1 banana and 1 orange Lunch: brown rice and steak Snack 2: yogurt and cookies Dinner: brown rice and fish, 3 cups of vegetables	Upper body day: 7 sets of push-ups, 10-20 reps 5 sets of tricep push-ups, 10-20 reps 5 sets of tricep dips, 10-20 reps Rest interval: 45 seconds to a minute

Sunday	Breakfast: 4 cups of cereal with milk Snack 1: 3 cups of fruits Lunch: noodles and 2 cups of vegetables Snack 2: a fistful of mixed nuts Dinner: chicken and rice burritos, 3 cups of vegetables	Abdominal day: 6 sets of scissors, 30 seconds 6 sets of sit-ups, 10-25 reps 6 sets of overhead raises, 15-20 reps Rest interval: 40 seconds
Monday	Breakfast: 4 packets of oatmeal with milk Snack 1: a fistful of almonds and 2 cups of vegetables Lunch: turkey-and-cheese sandwiches Snack 2: 3 cups of fruits Dinner: brown rice and fish, 3 cups of vegetables	Leg day: 6 sets of jumps, 8-10 reps 6 sets of glute-ups, 20-25 reps 5 sets of squats, 15-25 reps 5 sets of wall chair, 30 seconds Rest interval: 1 minute
Tuesday	Breakfast: 5-small-egg omelet and milk Snack 1: 3 cups of broccoli and milk Lunch: ham-and-jelly sandwiches Snack 2: 2 cups of fruits Dinner: steak and rice burritos, 3 cups of vegetables	Upper body day: 6 sets of push-ups, 10-20 reps 6 sets of tricep push-ups, 10-20 reps 6 sets of tricep dips, 10-20 reps Rest interval: 45 seconds to a minute

Wednesday	Breakfast: 3-large-egg omelet and milk Snack 1: 3 cups of fruit salad Lunch: peanut butter sandwich (no jelly) Snack 2: 3 cups of vegetables Dinner: brown rice and fish, 3 cups of vegetables	Rest day!
Thursday	Breakfast: 4 cups of cereal with milk Snack 1: 3 cups of vegetables Lunch: turkey-and-jelly sandwiches and 3 cups of vegetables Snack 2: 3 cups of fruit salad Dinner: fast food of your choice!	Extra rest day!
Friday	Breakfast: 3-large-egg omelet and milk Snack 1: fistful of mixed nuts Lunch: noodles and grilled chicken Snack 2: 3 cups of fruit salad Dinner: noodles and 2 cups of broccoli	Abdominal day: 6 sets of scissors, 10-20 seconds 6 sets of sit-ups, 10-25 reps 6 sets of overhead raises, 5-15 reps Rest interval: 40 seconds
Saturday	Breakfast: 4 cups of cereal with milk Snack 1: 3 cups of vegetables with orange juice Lunch: turkey-and-jelly sandwiches Snack 2: 3 cups of fruit salad Dinner: chicken and rice burritos, 3 cups of vegetables	Leg day: 5 sets of squats, 15-25 reps 5 sets of glute-ups, 20-25 reps 5 sets of jumps, 8-10 reps 5 sets of wall chair, 30 seconds Rest interval: 1 minute

Two-Week Plan, Strength Training
(Body-Weight Exercises): Advanced Level

Day	Nutrition Plan	Workout Plan
Sunday	Breakfast: 7 slices of french toast and milk Snack 1: 3 cups of fruits Lunch: pasta and grilled chicken Snack 2: 4 cups of vegetables Dinner: pasta and steak, 3 cups of vegetables	Upper body day: 10 sets of push-ups, 25 plus reps 8 sets of tricep push-ups, 20 plus reps 8 sets of tricep dips, 20 plus reps Rest interval: 1 minute
Monday	Breakfast: 5 cups of cereal with milk Snack 1: 4 cups of vegetables with juice Lunch: turkey-and-jelly sandwiches Snack 2: 4 cups of fruit salad Dinner: brown rice with fish, 3 cups of vegetables	Abdominal day: 7 sets of scissors, 1 minute 7 sets of sit-ups, 30 plus reps 10 sets of overhead raises, 20 plus reps Rest interval: 1 minute
Tuesday	Breakfast: 5 cups of cereal with milk Snack 1: 3 cups of vegetables Lunch: turkey-and-cheese sandwiches Snack 2: 2 cups of fruit salad and yogurt Dinner: fast food of your choice!	Leg day: 7 sets of squats, 30 plus reps 7 sets of glute-ups, 30 plus reps 10 sets of jumps, 10 plus reps 7 sets of wall chair, 1 minute Rest interval: 1 minute

Wednesday	Breakfast: 5-large-egg omelet and milk Snack 1: 4 cups of fruit salad Lunch: 2 peanut butter sandwiches (no jelly) Snack 2: 4 cups of vegetables Dinner: brown rice and fish, 3 cups of vegetables	Rest day! Enjoy your only rest day of the week!
Thursday	Breakfast: 6 packets of oatmeal with milk Snack 1: a handful of almonds and yogurt Lunch: turkey-and-cheese sandwiches and 3 cups of vegetables Snack 2: 4 cups of fruits or fruit salad Dinner: chicken and rice burritos, 4 cups of vegetables	Upper body day: 8 sets of tricep dips, 20 plus reps 8 sets of tricep push-ups, 20 plus reps 10 sets of push-ups, 25 plus reps Rest interval: 1 minute
Friday	Breakfast: 4-large-egg omelet with 2 cups of vegetables Snack 1: 2 bananas and 2 oranges Lunch: white rice and steak Snack 2: milk and cookies Dinner: brown rice and grilled chicken, 3 cups of vegetables	Abdominal day: 10 sets of scissors, 1 minute 7 sets of sit-ups, 30 plus reps 7 sets of overhead raises, 20 plus reps Rest interval: 1 minute

Saturday	Breakfast: 4-medium-sized-egg omelet and milk Snack 1: 3 medium-sized bananas Lunch: 2 turkey-and-cheese sandwiches Snack 2: 4 cups of vegetables Dinner: brown rice and fish, 3 cups of vegetables	Leg day: 10 sets of jumps, 10 plus reps 7 sets of squats, 30 plus reps 7 sets of glute-ups, 30 plus reps 7 sets of wall chair, 1 minute Rest interval: 1 minute
Sunday	Breakfast: 7 slices of french toast Snack 1: 3 medium-sized bananas Lunch: 2 turkey-and-cheese sandwiches Snack 2: 4 cups of vegetables with orange juice Dinner: brown rice with fish and 3 cups of vegetables	Upper body day: 8 sets of tricep dips, 20 plus reps 8 sets of tricep push-ups, 20 plus reps 10 sets of push-ups, 25 plus reps Rest interval: 1 minute
Monday	Breakfast: 5-small-egg omelet and milk Snack 1: 2 cups of fruits Lunch: brown rice and 3 cups of broccoli Snack 2: milk and cookies Dinner: noodles and steak, 3 cups of vegetables	Abdominal day: 10 sets of sit-ups, 30 plus reps 10 sets of overhead raises, 20 plus reps 8 sets of scissors, 1 minute Rest interval: 1 minute

Tuesday	Breakfast: 5-small-egg omelet and milk Snack 1: 3 cups of fruits Lunch: noodles and steak and 3 cups of vegetables Snack 2: fistful of mixed nuts and milk Dinner: brown rice with fish and 3 cups of vegetables	Leg day: 6 sets of jumps, 10 plus reps 8 sets of squats, 30 plus reps 8 sets of glute-ups, 30 plus reps 8 sets of wall chair, 1 minute Rest interval: 1 minute
Wednesday	Breakfast: 6 packets of oatmeal with milk Snack 1: fistful of almonds Lunch: ham-and-jelly sandwich with 3 cups of fruits Snack 2: 3 cups of vegetables Dinner: steak and rice burritos and 3 cups of vegetables	Rest day!
Thursday	Breakfast: 5 cups of cereal with milk Snack 1: 2 cups of fruits Lunch: pasta and grilled chicken and yogurt Snack 2: 3 cups of vegetables Dinner: pasta and steak, 3 cups of vegetables	Abdominal day: 8 sets of scissors, 1 minute 8 sets of sit-ups, 30 plus reps 8 sets of overhead raises, 20 plus reps Rest interval: 1 minute

Friday	Breakfast: 5 cups of cereal with milk Snack 1: 3 cups of fruit salad Lunch: turkey-and-cheese sandwiches and yogurt Snack 2: 2 cups of vegetables with a mango (in season) or any large fruit Dinner: fast food of your choice!	Upper body day: 8 sets of tricep dips, 20 plus reps 8 sets of tricep push-ups, 20 plus reps 8 sets of push-ups, 25 plus reps Rest interval: 1 minute
Saturday	Breakfast: 5-medium-egg omelet and milk Snack 1: 2 apples and yogurt Lunch: brown rice and 3 cups of broccoli Snack 2: 2 cups of fruits Dinner: noodles and steak, 3 cups of vegetables	Leg day: 10 sets of jumps, 10 plus reps 10 sets of squats, 30 plus reps 6 sets of glute-ups, 30 plus reps 6 sets of wall chair, 1 minute Rest interval: 1 minute

Two-Week Plan, Distance Running: Beginner Level

Day	Nutrition Plan	Workout Plan
Sunday	Breakfast: 1-large-egg omelet and milk Snack 1: 2 cups of fruits and yogurt Lunch: turkey and cream cheese bagel Snack 2: 2 cups of vegetables Dinner: pasta and turkey meatballs, 3 cups of vegetables	Run any route you please for 15 minutes with an abdominal session halfway. Abdominal session: 2 sets of overhead raises, 2 sets of scissors, 2 sets of sit-ups
Monday	Breakfast: 2 cups of cereal with milk Snack 1: 2 cups of fruits Lunch: brown rice and steak, 2 cups of vegetables Snack 2: a fistful of almonds and yogurt Dinner: brown rice with fish, 3 cups of vegetables	Rest day!
Tuesday	Breakfast: 1-small-egg omelet with two slices of bread and milk Snack 1: 2 cups of fruit salad Lunch: steak and pasta Snack 2: 4 cups of vegetables Dinner: any fast food of your choice!	15-minute run on hills with a friend
Wednesday	Breakfast: 3 packets of oatmeal with milk Snack 1: a bowl of fruits Lunch: turkey-and-cheese sandwich, 3 cups of vegetables Snack 2: milk and a slice of bread with jelly spread Dinner: steak and rice burritos, 3 cups of vegetables	2-3 miles at medium intensity on a level ground

Thursday	Breakfast: 3 packets of oatmeal with milk Snack 1: milk and 1 cup of fruits Lunch: turkey-and-cheese sandwich with two slices of whole wheat bread spread with pasta sauce Snack 2: fistful of mixed nuts Dinner: pasta with fish and 3 cups of vegetables	Rest day!
Friday	Breakfast: 2 cups of cereal with milk Snack 1: handful of almonds with 1 cup of vegetables Lunch: pasta and steak, 2 cups of vegetables Snack 2: 2 cups of fruits and yogurt Dinner: brown rice with fish, 3 cups of vegetables	1-2 miles at a jogging pace on a level ground
Saturday	Breakfast: 3 cups of cereal with milk Snack 1: 2 cups vegetables Lunch: ham-and-cheese sandwich, 2 cups of vegetables Snack 2: 2 cups of fruits and yogurt Dinner: chicken and rice burritos, 3 cups of vegetables	Rest day!
Sunday	Breakfast: 3 packets of oatmeal with milk Snack 1: 2 cups of vegetables Lunch: peanut butter sandwich (no jelly) Snack 2: 2 cups of fruits Dinner: brown rice with fish, 3 cups of vegetables	Run any route you please for 20 minutes. Side note: Listen to some tunes when you run! You won't be bored! ^_^

Monday	Breakfast: 2-small-egg omelet and milk Snack 1: 2 cups of fruits Lunch: turkey-and-cheese sandwich, 4 cups of vegetables Snack 2: 2 cups of vegetables Dinner: fast food of your choice!	Rest day!
Tuesday	Breakfast: 2 cups of cereal with milk Snack 1: 3 cups of fruits Lunch: chicken and rice burritos, 4 cups of vegetables Snack 2: 2 cups of vegetables Dinner: noodles with fish and 1 cup of broccoli	1-3 miles at an easy jogging pace in the mountains
Wednesday	Breakfast: 1-small-egg omelet and 1 cup of cereal with milk Snack 1: 1 orange and yogurt Lunch: noodles and 1 cup of broccoli Snack 2: milk and cookies Dinner: pasta with fish and 3 cups of vegetables	Hit 1-2 miles at high intensity.
Thursday	Breakfast: 3 packets of oatmeal with milk Snack 1: 2 cups of fruits Lunch: brown rice with fish and 1 cup of broccoli Snack 2: handful of walnuts and milk Dinner: pasta and turkey meatballs and 3 cups of vegetables	Rest day! Enjoy it!

Friday	Breakfast: 1-large-egg omelet and milk Snack 1: 2 cups of grapes and yogurt Lunch: fast food of your choice! Snack 2: 2 cups of fruit salad Dinner: pasta and grilled chicken, 3 cups of vegetables	Hit 3 miles at medium intensity. Side note: You should be able to do the run within 30 to 45 minutes.
Saturday	Breakfast: 3 slices of french toast and milk Snack 1: a handful of mixed nuts and milk Lunch: brown rice and 2 cups of vegetables Snack 2: 2 cups of fruits Dinner: steak and rice burritos, 3 cups of vegetables	Rest day!

Two-Week Plan, Distance Running: Intermediate Level

Day	Nutrition Plan	Workout Plan
Sunday	Breakfast: 4 slices of french toast and milk Snack 1: a handful of mixed nuts and yogurt Lunch: brown rice with fish and 2 cups of vegetables Snack 2: 2 cups of fruits Dinner: chicken and rice burritos, 3 cups of vegetables	Run any route you please for 30 minutes with an abdominal session halfway. Abdominal session: 3 sets of overhead raises, 3 sets of scissors, 3 sets of sit-ups
Monday	Breakfast: 2-large-egg omelet and milk Snack 1: 3 cups of fruit salad Lunch: pasta and grilled chicken, 3 cups of vegetables Snack 2: 3 cups of vegetables Dinner: fast food of your choice!	Run on hills for 30 minutes at medium intensity. Try to get in the 2.5- to 3.5-mile range.
Tuesday	Breakfast: 3-small-egg omelet and 1 cup of cereal with milk Snack 1: 3 cups of fruits Lunch: noodles and 2 cups of vegetables Snack 2: milk and cookies Dinner: pasta and turkey meatballs and 3 cups of vegetables	40-minute light run in the suburbs You should be able to hit at least 3 miles.

Wednesday	Breakfast: 3 cups of cereal with milk Snack 1: 3 cups of vegetables Lunch: noodles and turkey meatballs, 2 cups of vegetables Snack 2: 2 cups of fruits and yogurt Dinner: steak and rice burritos and 3 cups of vegetables	Rest day!
Thursday	Breakfast: 5 packets of oatmeal with milk Snack 1: fistful of almonds and yogurt Lunch: 2 turkey-and-cheese sandwiches, 3 cups of vegetables Snack 2: 2 cups of fruits Dinner: brown rice with fish and 2 cups of broccoli	Rest day!
Friday	Breakfast: 3-medium-egg omelet with milk Snack 1: handful of mixed nuts and milk Lunch: 2 ham-and-cheese sandwiches, 3 cups of vegetables Snack 2: 3 cups of fruit salad Dinner: brown rice and steak, 3 cups of vegetables	20-minute intense run Run wherever you want. Try to get into the 2- to 3-mile range.

Saturday	Breakfast: 5 slices of french toast with milk Snack 1: 3 cups of vegetables Lunch: peanut butter and jelly sandwich, 4 cups of vegetables Snack 2: 2 medium-sized bananas and yogurt Dinner: brown rice with fish, and 3 cups of vegetables	50-minute light run Try to get in the 4- to 6-mile range.
Sunday	Breakfast: 4 slices of french toast and milk Snack 1: 3 cups of berries Lunch: 2 chicken and rice burritos and 2 cups of vegetables Snack 2: yogurt and cookies Dinner: brown rice with fish, and 3 cups of vegetables	35-minute run at medium intensity on hills Try to cover at least 3 miles.
Monday	Breakfast: 5 packets of cereal with milk Snack 1: 3 cups of grapes Lunch: 2 ham-and-cheese sandwiches, 2 cups of vegetables Snack 2: fistful of mixed nuts Dinner: noodles with fish, 3 cups of vegetables	Rest day!

Tuesday	Breakfast: 5-small-egg omelet and milk Snack 1: 3 small bananas Lunch: 2 steak and rice burritos, 4 cups of vegetables Snack 2: 1 cup of yogurt with orange juice Dinner: noodles with fish and 2 cups of broccoli	40-minute run at medium intensity in the hills Run with a partner so that you will be motivated to push through the hills.
Wednesday	Breakfast: 5 packets of oatmeal with milk Snack 1: 2 fruits Lunch: 2 chicken and rice burritos, 3 cups of vegetables Snack 2: yogurt and 4 cups of vegetables Dinner: fast food of your choice!	Go for an easy jog for 15 minutes. Today is a recovery day from yesterday's grueling workout.
Thursday	Breakfast: 5 slices of french toast and milk Snack 1: 2 cups of fruit salad Lunch: 2 turkey-and-cheese sandwiches, 3 cups of vegetables Snack 2: fistful of mixed nuts and milk Dinner: brown rice with fish, 3 cups of vegetables	Rest day!

Friday	Breakfast: 3-large-egg omelet and milk Snack 1: 1 cup of yogurt, 1 cup of fruits Lunch: 2 turkey-and-cheese sandwiches and 3 cups of vegetables Snack 2: a handful of mixed nuts Dinner: brown rice with fish and 3 cups of vegetables	30-minute run at medium intensity with an abdominal session halfway Abdominal session: 4 sets of overhead raises, 3 sets of scissors, 3 sets of sit-ups
Saturday	Breakfast: 5 slices of french toast and milk Snack 1: 3 cups of fruit salad Lunch: 2 turkey-and-jelly sandwiches and 2 cups of vegetables Snack 2: fistful of mixed nuts and glass of milk Dinner: pasta with fish and 4 cups of vegetables	50-minute long run at medium intensity on a level ground

Two-Week Plan, Distance Running: Advanced Level

Day	Nutrition Plan	Workout Plan
Sunday	Breakfast: 4 slices of french toast and milk Snack 1: 4 cups of fruit salad Lunch: 2 ham-and-jelly sandwiches, 2 cups of vegetables Snack 2: fistful of mixed nuts and glass of milk Dinner: pasta with fish and 4 cups of vegetables	Run on hills for 45 minutes at medium intensity. Try to cover the 4- to 6-mile range.
Monday	Breakfast: 5-large-egg omelet and milk Snack 1: handful of mixed nuts and 2 cups of fruits Lunch: 2 turkey-and-cheese sandwiches, 3 cups of vegetables Snack 2: yogurt Dinner: brown rice and grilled chicken and 4 cups of vegetables	25-minute intense run with abdominal session halfway Abdominal session: 4 sets of overhead raises, 4 sets of scissors, 4 sets of sit-ups Try to cover at least 2.5 miles.
Tuesday	Breakfast: 5 slices of french toast and milk Snack 1: 3 cups of vegetable salad Lunch: 2 turkey-and-cheese sandwiches Snack 2: 2 cups of fruits, yogurt Dinner: brown rice with fish, 4 cups of vegetables	Rest day!

Wednesday	Breakfast: 4 cups of cereal with milk Snack 1: 3 cups of fruits Lunch: 2 ham-and-jelly sandwiches, 2 cups of yogurt Snack 2: 3 cups of vegetables Dinner: noodles and grilled chicken, 4 cups of vegetables	70-minute long run at medium intensity on a level ground Try to cover at least 6 miles.
Thursday	Breakfast: 4 cups of cereal with milk Snack 1: 2 cups of vegetables Lunch: 2 ham-and-cheese sandwiches, 2 cups of vegetables Snack 2: 2 cups of vegetables and 1 cup of yogurt Dinner: noodles with fish and 3 cups of vegetables	Go for an easy 20-minute jog. Today is a recovery day from yesterday's long workout.
Friday	Breakfast: 4 cups of cereal with milk Snack 1: 3 cups of vegetables Lunch: 2 steak and rice burritos, 2 cups of fruit Snack 2: 1 cup of fruit salad, 3 cups of vegetables Dinner: fast food of your choice	Rest day!
Saturday	Breakfast: 6-small-egg omelet and milk Snack 1: 3 cups of fruit salad Lunch: pasta with fish and 2 cups of broccoli Snack 2: fistful of mixed nuts, 1 cup of yogurt Dinner: 3 chicken and rice burritos, 3 cups of vegetables	50-minute run at medium intensity in the hills

Sunday	Breakfast: 5-large-egg omelet and milk Snack 1: milk and cookies Lunch: pasta and turkey meatballs and 2 cups of vegetables Snack 2: 3 cups of fruit salad Dinner: pasta with fish and 4 cups of vegetables	60-minute long run at medium intensity on a level ground Try to cover at least 6 miles.
Monday	Breakfast: 5 slices of french toast with 1 cup of broccoli Snack 1: 3 cups of berries Lunch: 3 chicken and rice burritos and 2 cups of yogurt Snack 2: 2 cups of vegetables Dinner: brown rice with fish and 4 cups of vegetables	20-minute intense run in the hills
Tuesday	Breakfast: 5 slices of french toast with orange juice Snack 1: 3 cups of fruits Lunch: pasta and grilled chicken, 2 cups of yogurt Snack 2: 1 cup of plain pasta with 3 cups of broccoli Dinner: brown rice with fish and 3 cups of vegetables	Rest day!

Wednesday	Breakfast: 4 cups of cereal with milk Snack 1: 2 cups of fruits Lunch: 2 ham-and-jelly sandwiches, 3 cups of vegetables Snack 2: fistful of mixed nuts and 2 cups of yogurt Dinner: pasta with fish and 2 cups of vegetable salad	30-minute light run Try to cover 3 miles.
Thursday	Breakfast: 7-small-egg omelet and milk Snack 1: 2 cups of fruits or yogurt Lunch: 2 turkey-and-jelly sandwiches, 3 cups of vegetables Snack 2: fistful of almonds and 1 cup of yogurt Dinner: noodles with chicken and 3 cups of vegetables	70-minute long run at medium intensity on a level ground Try to cover at least 6 miles.
Friday	Breakfast: 4 slices of french toast and milk Snack 1: 3 cups of fruits Lunch: 2 chicken and rice burritos, 3 cups of vegetables Snack 2: 2 cups of yogurt Dinner: pasta with fish and 3 cups of vegetables	Rest day!
Saturday	Breakfast: 4-medium-sized-egg omelet and milk Snack 1: 2 cup of fruits Lunch: 2 steak and rice burritos, 4 cups of vegetables Snack 2: 3 cups of vegetables, 2 cups of yogurt Dinner: fast food of your choice!	30-minute intense hill run This is an extremely challenging workout. Be prepared for it. Try to cover at least 3.5 miles.

Two-Week Plan, Sprinting/Strength Training/ Distance Running/Cross-Training: Beginner Level

Day	Nutrition Plan	Workout Plan
Sunday	Breakfast: 4 slices of french toast and milk Snack 1: 2 cups of grapes Lunch: ham-and-cheese sandwich, 1 cup of yogurt Snack 2: 2 cups of broccoli Dinner: steak and rice burritos, 3 cups of vegetables	5 × 100 meter sprints 75% top speed Rest interval between sprints: 1 minute
Monday	Breakfast: 3-small-egg omelet with milk Snack 1: fistful of mixed nuts Lunch: turkey-and-jelly sandwich, 1 cup of yogurt Snack 2: 2 cups of vegetables Dinner: brown rice with fish, 3 cups of vegetables	Rest day!
Tuesday	Breakfast: 2 cups of cereal with milk Snack 1: 2 cups of fruits Lunch: pasta and grilled chicken Snack 2: 2 cups of vegetable salad Dinner: pasta and steak, 3 cups of vegetables	3 sets of tricep dips, 5-10 reps 3 sets of tricep push-ups, 5-10 reps 3 sets of push-ups, 5-10 reps Rest interval between sets: 30 seconds

Wednesday	Breakfast: 3 packets of oatmeal with milk Snack 1: fistful of mixed nuts and 1 cup of yogurt Lunch: pasta with fish and 1 cup of broccoli Snack 2: milk and cookies Dinner: noodles and grilled chicken and 3 cups of vegetables	Rest day!
Thursday	Breakfast: 2 cups of cereal with milk Snack 1: 2 cups of vegetable salad Lunch: chicken and rice burritos, 1 cup of yogurt Snack 2: 3 tangerines Dinner: noodles with fish, 3 cups of vegetables	1-2 miles at a jogging pace on a level ground
Friday	Breakfast: 2-large-egg omelet and milk Snack 1: 2 cups of fruit salad Lunch: chicken and rice burritos, 2 cups of vegetables Snack 2: fistful of walnuts Dinner: fast food of your choice!	Rest day!
Saturday	Breakfast: 1-large-egg omelet and milk Snack 1: 2 cups of fruit salad Lunch: white rice and grilled chicken and 2 cups of vegetables Snack 2: a handful of almonds Dinner: pasta with fish and 3 cups of vegetables	Run any route you please for 20 minutes. Side note: Listen to some tunes when you run! You won't be bored! ^_^

Sunday	Breakfast: 2 cups of cereal with milk Snack 1: milk and cookies Lunch: white rice and steak and 2 cups of yogurt Snack 2: fistful of mixed nuts and milk Dinner: pasta with fish and 3 cups of vegetables	1 lap (set) of UCLAs
Monday	Breakfast: 2 cups of oatmeal with milk Snack 1: 2 cups of fruits Lunch: white rice and steak, 2 cups of vegetables Snack 2: 2 cups of vegetables Dinner: noodles and grilled chicken, 2 cups of vegetables	3 sets of sit-ups, 5-10 reps 3 sets of scissors, 10-20 seconds 4 sets of overhead raises, 5-15 reps Rest interval between sets: 40 seconds
Tuesday	Breakfast: 4 slices of french toast and milk Snack 1: 2 oranges or apples Lunch: brown rice and steak, 2 cups of vegetables Snack 2: 1 cup of yogurt Dinner: brown rice with fish and 3 cups vegetables	Rest day!
Wednesday	Breakfast: 2 slices of french toast and milk Snack 1: 2 cups of grapes Lunch: brown rice and steak, 1 cup of yogurt Snack 2: 2 cups of vegetable salad Dinner: brown rice with fish and 3 cups of vegetables	Hit 2 miles at medium intensity. Side note: You should be able to do the run within 20 to 30 minutes.

Thursday	Breakfast: 2 cups of cereal with milk Snack 1: 2 apples Lunch: brown rice with fish and 1 cup of broccoli Snack 2: 3 cups of vegetables Dinner: fast food of your choice!	3 sets of tricep dips, 5-10 reps 3 sets of tricep push-ups, 5-10 reps 4 sets of push-ups, 5-10 reps Rest interval between sets: 30 seconds
Friday	Breakfast: 3 slices of french toast with milk Snack 1: 2 oranges Lunch: peanut butter and jelly sandwich, 2 cups of vegetables Snack 2: 1 cup of broccoli and 1 cup of yogurt Dinner: brown rice with fish and 3 cups of vegetables	Rest day!
Saturday	Breakfast: 2 cups of cereal with milk Snack 1: 2 cups of fruits Lunch: peanut butter sandwich (no jelly) Snack 2: 2 cups of vegetable salad Dinner: chicken and rice burritos and 3 cups of vegetables	Rest day!

The reader can come up with his or her own cross-training workout plans for intermediate—and advanced-level workouts. Since you have completed reading my guide, go formulate your workouts. Get fit and lead a healthy lifestyle!

References

1. Carr, Gerry A. 1991. *Fundamentals of Track and Field*. 2nd ed. Leisure Press.
2. *Wikipedia*. "Dynamic Stretching." *Wikimedia Foundation*. March 8, 2012. Web. 28 Aug. 2012. http://en.wikipedia.org/wiki/Dynamic_stretching.
3. Douglas, Scott, and Amby Burfoot. 2011. *The Little Red Book of Running*. New York: Skyhorse.
4. Burfoot, Amby. 2012. *Runner's World Training Journal: 52 Weeks of Motivation, Training Tips, Nutrition Advice, and Much More for Every Kind of Runner*. New York: Rodale Press.
5. Pierce, Bill James, Ray Moss, and Scott Murr. 2012. *Run Less, Run Faster: Become a Faster, Stronger Runner with the Revolutionary 3-runs-a-week Training Program*. Emmaus, PA: Rodale Press.
6. Delavier, Frédéric. 2001. *Strength Training Anatomy*. 3rd ed. Champaign, IL: Human Kinetics.
7. Schwarzenegger, Arnold, and Bill Dobbins. 1998. *The New Encyclopedia of Modern Bodybuilding*. New York: Simon & Schuster.
8. "What Is Insomnia?" December 2011. National Heart Lung and Blood Institute (NHLBI, NIH) 13 Web. 28 Aug. 2012. http://www.nhlbi.nih.gov/health/health-topics/topics/inso.
9. Colbert, Don. 2007. *The Seven Pillars of Health*. Lake Mary, FL: Siloam.
10. Scott, Elizabeth. August 27, 2012. "Caffeine, Stress and Your Health: Is Caffeine Your Friend or Your Foe?" About.com Stress Management. About.com Guide. Web. September 3, 2012. http://stress.about.com/od/stresshealth/a/caffeine.htm.

11. Nordqvist, Christian. January 26, 2012. "What Is Nicotine?" *Medical News Today*. MediLexicon International. Web. September 3, 2012. http://www.medicalnewstoday.com/articles/240820.php.

12. Inlander, Charles B., and Jim Punkre. 1994. *Test Yourself for Maximum Health*. Allentown, PA: People's Medical Society.

13. Smith, Mike. 2005. *High Performance Sprinting*. Ramsbury: Crowood.

14. Chopra, Deepak. 1994. *Perfect Weight*. New York: Quantum Publications.

15. Ryan, Monique. 2007. *Sports Nutrition for Endurance Athletes*. Boulder, CO: VeloPress.

16. Fitzgerald, Matt. 2009. *Racing Weight*. Boulder, CO: VeloPress.

17. Harper, Bob, and Greg Critser. 2012. *The Skinny Rules*. London: Ballantine.

18. Mcgee, Bobby, and Mark Plaatjes. 2009. *Run Workouts for Runners and Triathletes*. Boulder, CO: VeloPress.

19. Goodman, Anthony A. "The Myths of Nutrition and Fitness." Lecture.

20. Goodman, Anthony A. "Lifelong Health: Achieving Optimum Well-Being at Any Age." Lecture.

21. Hodgkin, Dean. "Physiology and Fitness." Lecture.

22. Distel, Dara. March 29, 2011. "Musculature Anatomy Chart." Digital image. Dara Distel Fitness. Dara Distel Fitness. Web. January 6, 2013. http://daradistelfitness.com/human-body/muscle-diagram.

23. Gruber, Karl. August 2, 2010. "Track Training Techniques." Livestrong. com. Livestrong Web.

24. For nutritional information, refer to USDA government website: www. choosemyplate.gov.

Notes

Notes

CPSIA information can be obtained
at www.ICGtesting.com
Printed in the USA
LVHW090334141218
600438LV00002B/168/P